CAN HURT MORE
YOUR LOOKS

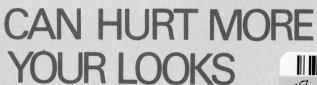

Atherosclerosis

Atherosclerosis is the deposit of fatty material in the lining of the arterial wall. It can result in rupture of the blood vessel or in narrowing of these vessels, which may lead to stroke or heart attack. Sudies show that there is a marked increase in the occurrence of atherosclerosis in overweight people.

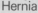

Heart

As one gains weight, the heart must work harder to supply nutrients to all tissues of the body. The greater the body mass, the greater the strain on the heart. There is a higher incidence of heart disease in people who are overweight.

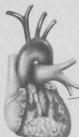

Hernia

Certain types of hernias, involving displacement of the upper part of the stomach into the chest cavity, are more prevalent in overweight individuals than in those of normal weight.

The omentum

Many overweight people assume that their "pot-bellied" appearance is due not to fat but to a protruding stomach. Actually, their shape is only partially due to the accumulation of fat under the skin; most of the bulge results from fat accumulated within the abdominal cavity—in the omentum.

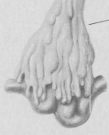

Adipose tissue

Adipose (fat) tissue is composed of cells which are highly elastic and contain varying amounts of fatty deposits acquired via the bloodstream. The tissue is situated throughout the body—under the skin in protective pacs covering vital organs, and in association with muscles. Excessive fat deposits are found in virtually all soft tissues and organs in overweight people. The degree of overweight depends upon the number of fat cells present and the amount of fat they contain. In the course of weight reduction, fat cell volume is decreased, but the number of fat cells remains constant.

Baby fat

Baby fat is not cute. When excess weight is gained during childhood, the number of fat cells in the body increases. Since the fat cells developed in childhood remain throughout life, it becomes exceedingly difficult to lose weight as an adult.

Dr. Wechsler's

NEW

YOU

DIET

Dr. Wechsler's

NEW YOU DIET

DR. ARNOLD WECHSLER

Citadel Press   Secaucus, N.J.

First Edition
Copyright © 1978 by Arnold Wechsler
All rights reserved
Published by Citadel Press
A division of Lyle Stuart Inc.
120 Enterprise Ave., Secaucus, N.J. 07094
In Canada: George J. McLeod Limited, Toronto
Manufactured in the United States of America

Library of Congress Cataloging in Publication Data

Wechsler, Arnold.
　　Dr. Wechsler's New you diet.
　　1.　Reducing diets.　2.　High-Protein diet.　I.　Title.
II.　Title:　New you diet.
RM222.2.W297　　　　　613.2′5　　　　78-17978
ISBN 0-8065-0630-X

CONTENTS

Dr. Wechsler's

NEW

YOU

DIET

Chapter 1
Hello...

My name is Arnold Wechsler and I'm a physician. I have practiced gynecological surgery at a large suburban hospital in Delaware County near Philadelphia. Twenty years ago, when I was beginning my practice, I helped found the hospital and became chairman of the Obs-Gyn Department. Although I'm no longer active in patient care at the hospital, I am still on its board of directors and chairman of the department.

I've never been a "diet" doctor and this is not just another diet book. I don't make any outrageous claims such as "You Can Lose Weight While You Sleep." I don't offer magic formulas. I don't even guarantee that you'll lose a fixed number of pounds in the first week or the first month.

My reasons for this are quite simple: My diet program is not a fad diet. It is based on the principle that effective weight control comes from treating the *total person*, not just one part of your body or one aspect of your personality. It is a simple, safe, commonsense approach that will help you for the rest of your life.

Best of all, you don't need to be a dietician or food chemist to understand it.

This book can give you—if you read and use it carefully—the information you need to make decisions about your personal weight problem and to do something about it. It will show you if you're eating wrong and why. It will, I believe, show you how to become a healthier you.

My diet approach has grown out of many years of practice with pregnant women. I succeeded in teaching them proper nutrition and successful weight control without confusion, calorie-counting, food lists and strange recipes. I did this by a practical method, one that I had used myself.

My personal experience with problem weight started when I was a resident. After months of eating nothing but starchy hospital cafeteria food, I woke up one morning to discover that there was twenty pounds too much of me.

So I created a diet that made sense to me. I restricted myself to one large meal a day, a meal made up entirely of high protein, low carbohydrate and low fat food. This wasn't the easiest diet in the world.

Like most Americans, I had an outrageous craving for sweets. There was a long period in my life when I wasn't comfortable without a glass of Coca-Cola in my hand. But I wanted to lose that extra weight, and I did—by using total will power. In other words, pure self-torture.

In case you're wondering how I've fared during the past twenty years, I am currently 5' 11" and weigh 160 pounds.

My feelings about the dangers of being overweight were greatly influenced—but by no means confined—by my work with pregnant women. Over the years I discovered that women who kept their weight gain within strict limits during pregnancy (usually 20-24 pounds) had fewer problems. Many women who gained excessive weight developed problems, both before and during delivery.

I prescribed for all of them a simple diet of protein (lean meat, fish or poultry), green and yellow leafy vegetables, and very little fat or starch. They were also directed to eat smaller meals, take prenatal vitamins and to exercise regularly. It was basically the same regimen I followed myself.

In medical school and during my residency, heavy emphasis was placed on the need for good nutrition as an integral part of good health. If a doctor treats a patient without being aware of the relationship between good nutrition and good health, he is giving an inadequate and incomplete service to that patient.

Good health requires good nutrition. That is what I mean by treating the *total person.*

Chapter 2

Let's Begin With You

Recently, you may have been confused and frightened by news reports about protein diets. This is unfortunate. Baseless accusations have been blown out of proportion by government agencies and the news media. Because of this, all protein food supplements are being tarred with the same brush.

I believe that the consumer should be protected. But I do not believe you should be driven crazy by erroneous accusations and incomplete evaluations. You deserve intelligent information and sensible nutritional knowledge, not the type of misinformation that is being passed around now.

That is exactly my purpose—to give you the right kind of information so you can make up your own mind about the type of weight control program you want and need. Protein is not a "poison." It is as important to your health as breathing itself.

I assume you've journeyed down the diet road before, probably several times. You've been buried under an avalanche of fad diets and weight reducing devices. You've probably tried a number of them and found that they don't work. Fad diets always promise much but deliver little.

I'm not going to offer you any fad diet magic, because when it comes to true and lasting weight control, magic doesn't exist. What I offer is better than magic, because it's real. If you're like most overweight people, it took years to get to where you are today. No one can lose the accumulation of years of hard eating in just a few weeks. Anyone who tells you that is not speaking truth.

With my diet approach, you can solve the problem of excess weight. It won't be easy but it will be effective and safe. Unlike many diets, it doesn't sacrifice good nutrition. A diet that emphasizes weight loss at any cost is not a good diet.

Permanent weight control is what you're really after. I can direct you to that goal.

My weight control method makes good nutritional sense and makes the most sense if you *really* want to solve the problem of excess weight. In these pages I'll share with you all the information you need to make your own decisions, calmly and safely.

Of prime importance, you will learn about nutrition and ways to control your weight that will be both *safe and successful.*

Chapter 3

The Sad State of Affairs

Recently, a widely known British character actor died unexpectedly. He once described himself as "a rather dashing figure, like Falstaff." He was pleased with his figure, one that objectively could only be described as massive! He was 5' 9" tall and weighed 280 pounds! His weight, he explained, was the result of his enthusiasm for cooking and his frequent visits to expensive restaurants.

His name was Sebastian Cabot, and he was fifty-nine when he died of a stroke. It was the second stroke for the actor in three years. He didn't die because of his or anyone else's cooking. He died because he ate too much of the wrong food. When he died, he was severely malnourished.

If you're overweight, you may never get the chance to play Falstaff on any stage except possibly the one that you set up in your own kitchen. Like Cabot, however, you run the very real risk of dying at an early age. Unless you possess his charm and dignity, people will treat you with embarrassed delicacy. You will not be described by your friends as a "dashing figure." You will be described as fat, obese, tubby or just plain gross. More than likely, you will be just plain miserable.

You are not alone.

Even though the data on overweight people in this country remains incomplete, among insured people—and who is better at compiling statistics than the insurance companies?—half of the men between thirty and thirty-nine are at least ten percent overweight and a

Desirable Body Weights

(The following are desirable weights for men and women over 25, graded according to body frame. These tables, prepared by the Metropolitan Life Insurance Company, are based on weights associated with the lowest mortality. The charts allow about 8 pounds for men's clothing and 4 pounds for women's. To arrive at the normal weight of girls 18 to 25, subtract 1 pound for each year under 25.)

Height (with shoes on)		MEN Weight in pounds, as ordinarily dressed including shoes and suit		
Feet	Inches	Small frame	Medium frame	Large frame
5	2	112–120	118–129	126–141
5	3	115–123	121–133	129–144
5	4	118–126	124–136	132–148
5	5	121–129	127–139	135–152
5	6	124–133	130–143	138–156
5	7	128–137	134–147	142–161
5	8	132–141	138–152	147–166
5	9	136–145	142–156	151–170
5	10	140–150	146–160	155–174
5	11	144–154	150–165	159–179
6	0	148–158	154–170	164–184
6	1	152–162	158–175	168–189
6	2	156–167	162–180	173–194
6	3	160–171	167–185	178–199
6	4	164–175	172–190	182–204

quarter of those are at least twenty percent overweight. After age fifty, the percentages increase dramatically. The statistics on women are about the same except that the percentage of overweight women over age fifty is significantly larger.

The saddest part of all these weight statistics are those for school children. One study in Massachusetts revealed that ten percent of the children tested were overweight.

Obesity is a major disease in this country and in western Europe. Unlike most diseases, however, it is self-inflicted. It is like going into a room and beating yourself with a chain.

Sebastian Cabot was, by almost any definition available, obese. As many as thirty percent of *all* Americans are in the same boat.

Height (with shoes on; 2-in heels)		WOMEN Weight in pounds, as ordinarily dressed, including shoes and dress		
Feet	Inches	Small frame	Medium frame	Large frame
4	10	92–98	96–107	104–119
4	11	94–101	98–110	106–122
5	0	96–104	101–113	109–125
5	1	99–107	104–116	112–128
5	2	102–110	107–119	115–131
5	3	105–113	110–122	118–134
5	4	108–116	113–126	121–138
5	5	111–119	116–130	125–142
5	6	114–123	120–135	129–146
5	7	118–127	124–139	133–150
5	8	122–131	128–143	137–154
5	9	126–135	132–147	141–158
5	10	130–140	136–151	145–163
5	11	134–144	140–155	149–168
6	0	138–148	144–159	153–173

According to these figures, Sebastian Cabot *should* have weighed no more than 170 pounds. Even giving him the benefit of the doubt by adding ten percent, he was still grossly overweight.

Obesity is a disease and one—unless it is the result of some severe metabolic dysfunction—that can be controlled. That is what this book is all about. It is not a song and dance routine nor a get-thin-quick scheme nor a magic wand you can wave in front of your refrigerator door to scare the fat cells away.

My method, if followed faithfully, can turn you into the person you want to be: thin, attractive and, most importantly, healthy.

The height and weight tables are good guides, but the easiest way to find out if you're overweight is simply to look at yourself. You've done this hundreds of times before and probably spent most of that time rationalizing your appearance. This time I want you to look at yourself objectively. No rationalizations!

Let's do it this way. First, find yourself a room with a full-length mirror. A full-length mirror, not one that reflects you only from the neck up. Now, close all the doors, all the curtains and turn out all the lights.

Take off all your clothes. Sounds sexy, doesn't it? It doesn't get better. It gets worse.

Here's where it gets worse. Turn on the lights! What do you see?

Who is that person gaping uncomfortably at you from the mirror?

If you're a woman, is it someone your lover will daydream about at work?

Are you someone who used to wear a forty regular and now has trouble squeezing himself into a forty-six wide?

What you see, unfortunately, is what you are now.

Don't tell yourself it's not so bad. I mean, with the right kind of dress or the right kind of coat you could look, well, almost acceptable. Nonsense! The problem is not what you wear, even though clothing manufacturers are falling all over themselves to provide you with those so-called mature styles. In reality they are manufacturing "fat sizes" and you're the only one they're making them for.

Take another good look at yourself. Try to remember what you looked like before you "filled out." How long has it taken you to get this way? Are you happy? Are you satisfied with yourself?

Of course not.

The next question you should ask is: Have I finally had enough of this foolishness? I trust that your answer is yes, or you would not have come to me for help.

Okay, now you can put your clothes back on.

Chapter 4

How You Got the Way You Are

The reason for all the fat clogging up the bedrooms and kitchens of the world is that we eat too much, we eat the wrong kinds of food and we don't exercise enough.

In post-industrial societies such as the United States and western Europe, we have made life easier for ourselves. We have also paid our dues for that development. We have conquered drudgery and we have developed prepared foods that have just about eliminated the art of cooking. Less work and very little exercise have become our way of life. We put more food into our mouths than we need and most of it is the wrong kind.

That food isn't going any place either. It stays in our bodies and turns into fat.

Food is fuel—energy. Food is gasoline for your body's engine. But your body has a limit as to how much fuel it can use. If we feed ourselves too much energy, our bodies will store the excess. Then we become fat.

The cost is enormous.

Fact: Overweight people are more susceptible to death from heart attacks, strokes, diabetes, gallstones, appendicitis and even accidents than people who maintain a reasonable weight.

It is also believed that these mortality figures have been grossly underestimated. The threat is actually much worse. It is interesting to note that one diet book, written years ago, stated the case plainly in its title *Why Die?*

Being fat isn't much fun, either. The public doesn't particularly like fat people. Studies done with children have shown that the obese child is almost universally disliked and discriminated against. Other studies, done with adults, showed an even wider range of discrimination. Doctors had extremely negative attitudes towards their overweight patients. Colleges were apt not to accept obese applicants. Overweight people were described as "ugly" and "weak willed."

This is because society puts great emphasis on appearance. It is, for better or worse, one of the primary ways in which we are judged as individuals. It may not be fair but it is a factor.

At one time, between the years 1500 and 1900, being fat was "in." Corpulence was considered a blessing and people cultivated their fat. They mistakenly thought that being fat was the same as being healthy. You, unfortunately, live in the twentieth century, when being fat is just being fat.

Today we are continually assaulted with images of good looking thin people. They're everywhere. Svelte models with too many teeth and shimmering hair sell us tires and deodorants. Athletic young men with razor haircuts and aquiline noses model for ads that suggest we can look like them.

Remember, only a model looks like a model.

A model is paid a large amount of money to look the way she does. She is surrounded by a retinue of hairdressers, masseurs, makeup men, directors, photographers and bodyguards. All of these people are paid to keep her the way she is. Nobody is going to pay you to lose weight. If you are like most people, you're going to have to do it completely on your own.

At the very same time television tells us what we should all look like, it also tempts us in the opposite direction. It shows you exactly what you're trying desperately to avoid: FOOD.

Pick any night of the week and turn on your television. What do you see?

You see sandwiches the size of Lithuania. You see desserts that look like the Matterhorn. You see pieces of cake that could sink an aircraft carrier. You hear somebody saying, "When I make a barbecue, I make a *Big Barbecue!*"

This caloric sideshow is repeated endlessly, night after night, week after week. What happens? You succumb to the repetition and your will power disappears. Like some primitive, you march into the kitchen, yank open the refrigerator door, and inhale the contents thereof.

Then you see some 105-pound model and you feel guilty. After flogging your conscience—"I will never eat again!"—you watch a few more Sara Lee commercials and the process is repeated.

Television may be bad for adults, but it is worse for children. You may have some notion of what's going on, but a child usually does not. The statisitics on television viewing by American children are more than staggering. They are absolutely mind-boggling.

An average child sees more than *20,000* commercials a year on television. Between the ages of three and eighteen, that child may see as many as *325,000* commercials. By the time he or she reaches college age, the average American child will have spent nearly *3,000* hours in front of the television set. In that length of

U.S. Recommended Daily Allowance (U.S.RDA)
(for use in nutrition labeling of foods, including foods that also are vitamin and mineral supplements)

	Adults and Children Over 4 Years of Age	Children Under 4 Years of Age	Infants Under 13 Months	Pregnant or Lactating Women
Protein	65 g*	28 g*	25 g*	65 g*
Vitamin A	5,000 IU	2,500 IU	2,500 IU	8,000 IU
Vitamin C	60 mg	40 mg	40 mg	60 mg
Thiamine	1.5 mg	0.7 mg	0.7 mg	1.7 mg
Riboflavin	1.7 mg	0.8 mg	0.8 mg	2.0 mg
Niacin	20 mg	9.0 mg	9.0 mg	20 mg
Calcium	1.0 g	0.8 g	0.8 g	1.3 g
Iron	18 mg	10 mg	10 mg	18 mg
Vitamin D	400 IU	400 IU	400 IU	400 IU
Vitamin E	30 IU	10 IU	10 IU	30 IU
Vitamin B_6	2.0 mg	0.7 mg	0.7 mg	2.5 mg
Folacin	0.4 mg	0.2 mg	0.2 mg	0.8 mg
Vitamin B_{12}	6 μg	3 μg	3 μg	8 μg
Phosphorus	1.0 g	0.8 g	0.8 g	1.3 g
Iodine	150 μg	70 μg	70 μg	150 μg
Magnesium	400 mg	200 mg	200 mg	450 mg
Zinc	15 mg	8 mg	8 mg	15 mg
Copper	2 mg	1 mg	1 mg	2 mg
Biotin	0.3 mg	0.15 mg	0.15 mg	0.3 mg
Pantothenic acid	10 mg	5 mg	5 mg	10 mg

* If protein efficiency ratio of protein is equal to or better than that of casein, U.S.RDA is 45 g for adults and pregnant or lactating women, 20 g for children under 4 years of age, and 18 g for infants.

SOURCE: The National Nutrition Consortium, Inc., with Ronald M. Deutsch: *Nutrition Labeling: How It Can Work for You.* Bethesda, Md.: National Nutrition Consortium, Inc., 1975. Based on *Federal Register.* Vol. 38, no. 13, part III, January 19, 1973.

time, the child could have attended college, graduated and probably gotten a Master's degree to boot.

And what do children see in these commercials? They see an enormous amount of nutritional misinformation. They see ads for breakfast cereals that are often more than fifty percent sugar and, they are told, these cereals will be giving them a "well balanced meal." Though the cereals are often fortified with vitamins and minerals, their main ingredient is sugar.

It would be very easy to blame television, magazines, newspapers, radio, movies or even your neighborhood supermarket for all this. They are certainly the convenient villains. But television—and the other modern media—was not invented in a social vacuum. Television is simply the most effective way to spread these self-destructive eating patterns.

In the western world—America and Europe—abundance is taken for granted. For many years it was taken as a sign from God that he liked what was going on down here. So we indulged ourselves.

We ate even when we weren't hungry. We created Thanksgiving Day and dedicated it to overeating. Here, we said, take a day off from work and stuff yourself silly. Expansion was the key word.

We used up our own resources—and the world's for that matter—with great abandon. Big cars, big houses and big cities. We were having a terrific time! When we began to wake up, we found out that things weren't all that terrific. What we got for our indulgence was an energy crisis, a housing shortage, urban blight and fat people.

Big, bigger, biggest, huge, humungous, gigantic—Fat, Fat, Fat! ! !

But these things can change.

And so can you.

Chapter 5

The Sugar Blues

Along with the problem of excess comes the problem of *what* we eat. If as a people we eat too much, we also eat too much of the wrong things.

Sugar, for instance.

At the beginning of the twentieth century, the average American consumed seventy-six pounds of refined sugar a year. Today we eat well over ninety-five pounds of sugar per person a year, and the quantity is rising.

What does sugar do for us? It's true that it provides energy, but energy can be gotten from more healthful sources. Sugar doesn't provide strength, vitamins, minerals or fiber. It doesn't even give you the feeling of being full. Aside from some quick energy, all it does is make you fat. If you eat enough of it, it will make you very fat. Your teeth will rot. You will be very fat *and* you will have rotten teeth.

Like narcotics, sugar creates an addiction—a constant, almost insatiable hunger for more sugar.

We also consume vast amounts of junk foods which, by the way, usually contain vast amounts of sugar. (Why do you think they call it *junk*?) We have candy bars, candy-coated breakfast cereals and soft drinks. Some of you are so far gone, you wouldn't know good food if it moved in next door.

You'd think we'd all be sick of junk food by now, but we're not.

We start as children with sugarized baby food. A number of child nutrition experts believe that this indoctrination of young children may be one of the major causes of obesity in adolescence and adulthood. The child gets used to the sweet taste and, as his or her desires become stronger, the parents succumb, buying the kids what they want: sugar. As they get older, the desire for sugarized food remains.

Here are some more consumption statistics that show just how bad our sugar addiction really is: According to the U.S. Department of Commerce, Americans ate 3,466,790,000 *pounds* of candy last year, approximately sixteen and a half *pounds per person*. That cost us about $2,912,000,000.

Partially in response to criticism, at least one major manufacturer of baby foods recently removed sugar from its products. The ironic thing is that sugar originally was added to baby food to please the parents, not the baby. The parents complained that the food wasn't sweet enough for *them!* So the manufacturers added sugar. Terrific!

Most obese children and teenagers are from families where at least one of the parents is obese. This should come as no surprise to you.

Our overconsumption of sugar isn't the only factor that contributes to our national weight problem. Our total food environment—what we eat and how we eat—has changed dramatically.

If both parents are fat, the child has a slim chance of

not being fat. It is much harder for those overweight children when they eventually grow into overweight adults to lose that excess fat.

The social patterns of the last hundred years—the nuclear family, shopping at the neighborhood grocer, eating three square meals a day—are gone.

Single adults are the fastest growing segment of our society. Our national birthrate is declining. More people eat out in restaurants than ever before. More often than not, they eat at fast food restaurants. The evening meal at home may be the only time family members see each other.

Primary foods—fresh produce—are no longer the mainstay of our diet. Taking their place are processed convenience foods. The reason for this change is obvious. People don't want to spend half a day cooking in the kitchen anymore. They want to be able to pull a package out of the freezer, stick it in the oven and presto—a full-blown meal.

We eat on the go, on the run and on our feet. We eat more snack foods. Snack foods may taste good (amazing what they can do with chemicals these days!) but they are not nutritious, just tasty and fattening.

Our obsession with convenience food is also leading to the disappearance of the corner grocer who often stocked fresh produce. Supermarkets, only twenty percent of the food stores in the United States right now, sell about three-quarters of the food purchased here. Because of the cost of storage and transportation, they stock packaged processed foods.

Lost in this maze of containers is the consumer who really has no choice. You have to eat and you have to shop, and most people, despite anything they have been told, will continue to buy what is most convenient.

And most fattening.

There are some changes. The expanding interest in natural foods is a good start. The rise in consumer awareness is another good sign.

You too can break out of these national food habits. You will if you want to.

Chapter 6
Bad Nutrition

Nutrition is a lot like the weather. Everyone is concerned about it, but nobody seems to be able to do very much about it. We know we need it, but we're not too sure how to get it. Unlike the weather, however, there is a lot that can be done about nutrition.

Good nutrition is ignored by most crash dieters because they are trapped in the clutches of a weight loss frenzy and don't want to hear about it. They want to lose weight yesterday, and good nutrition is the first thing they throw out the window. They have many excuses. It's too complex. It takes too much time. It has no bearing on weight loss. Blah, blah, blah.

You need not make the same mistake. Trying to divorce good nutrition from the problems of weight loss and weight control is a basic error in judgment, one that can prove dangerous to your mental and physical health.

Without good nutrition first and above everything else, weight loss and weight control are almost impossible to achieve and maintain.

If you're overweight, you have an unbalanced system.

Despite this, your body does the best it can. It changes and adapts. That doesn't mean it's happy with it. It isn't. If all the overweight bodies in the world could form a union, they would all go out on strike to protest unsafe working conditions.

In the book *Diet and Disease*, the authors (Cheraskin, Ringsdorf and Clark) point out that in economically developed countries like the United States, there has been an increase in total caloric intake, particularly those calories that come from refined sugar.

This increased consumption of sugar is deceptive. Very rarely do you sit around your living room snacking on teaspoons of sugar. Mostly it is hidden in other things, things we have literally taught ourselves to enjoy: a four-ounce piece of hard candy contains twenty tea-spoons of sugar; one slice of cherry pie contains ten; a glazed doughnut contains six; a half-cup of rice pudding contains five; an ice cream cone contains three and a half; a single chocolate bar contains almost three tea-spoons of sugar. (Each teaspoon of sugar equals fifteen calories!)

The problem doesn't stop there. While we've been increasing our consumption of sugar, we have also been increasing our consumption of fats—particularly satu-rated fats, cholesterol and salt.

There has also been a decrease in the consumption of some very basic nutrients, such as vitamins, minerals and protein. This is malnutrition—bad nutrition—as opposed to undernutrition, which is the major problem of Third World countries. They don't have enough to eat. In economically developed countries we have more than enough food, and our response to this abundance has been disastrous. We eat the things that do us the least amount of nutritional good. Then we complain about how bad we feel.

As the comic strip character Pogo remarked: "We have met the enemy and he is us."

This trend towards malnutrition is frightening. As more and more research is done, we find that there is a direct correlation between malnutrition and disease and aging.

For instance, a long term study in Norway showed that when the diets of pregnant women were nutritionally improved, stillbirths were cut down by one half, premature births decreased fifty percent, and infant mortality within the first year of life also declined substantially.

Certain mental disorders can be controlled with better nutrition. One study showed that when a group of men were not given an adequate amount of protein daily they became irritable and hard to get along with. Others problems ranging from simple headache to chronic insomnia may also be caused by malnutrition.

Now, obviously, good nutrition won't solve all your physical or emotional problems. Nor will it turn you into a perfect human being. But there is enough evidence available to prove that many diseases are affected by malnutrition. Whether they are actually caused by it is beside the point. The facts indicate that malnutrition makes these problems worse.

The list of these suspect ailments is endless: mental retardation, cancer, heart disease, infertility, impotence, loss of memory and concentration, skin diseases, cataracts, diabetes, stroke, arthritis, high blood pressure, digestive problems and even tuberculosis.

Oh yes, and obesity. Obesity reflects a severe lack of

Calorie Values of Some Common Snack Foods

Food	Weight gm.	Approximate measure	Calories
Beverages			
Carbonated, cola type	180	1 bottle, 6 ounces	70
Malted milk	405	1 regular (1½ cups)	420
Chocolate milk (made with skim milk)	250	1 cup	190
Cocoa	200	1 cup	235
Soda, vanilla ice cream	242	1 regular	260
Cake			
Angel food	40	2-inch sector	110
Cupcake, chocolate, iced	50	1 cake, 2¾ inches in diameter	185
Fruit cake	30	1 piece, 2 by 2 by ½ inch	115
Candy and Popcorn			
Butterscotch	15	3 pieces	60
Candy bar, plain	57	1 bar	295
Caramels	30	3 medium	120
Chocolate coated creams	30	2 average	130
Fudge	28	1 piece	115
Peanut brittle	30	1 ounce	125
Popcorn with oil added	14	1 cup	65
Cheese			
Camembert	28	1 ounce	85
Cheddar	28	1 ounce	105
Cream	28	1 ounce	105
Swiss (domestic)	28	1 ounce	105
Cookies			
Brownies	30	1 piece, 2 by 2 by ¾ inch	140
Cookies, plain and assorted	25	1 cooky, 3 inches in diameter	120

Crackers			
Cheese	18	5 crackers	85
Graham	14	2 medium	55
Saltines	16	4 crackers	70
Rye	13	2 crackers	45
Dessert type cream puff and Doughnuts			
Cream puff—custard filling	105	1 average	245
Doughnut, cake type, plain	32	1 average	125
Doughnut, jelly	65	1 average	225
Doughnut, raised	30	1 average	120

nutritional balance. This imbalance doesn't need to be gigantic. It can actually be very small. As one nutritionist pointed out, a healthy individual may eat as much as eight tons of food in the course of ten years. If only *five percent* of that food is retained rather than energized, that person would gain *eighty pounds*.

Admittedly, this litany of disease is a scare tactic. According to my plan, you should be recoiling in horror right about now. Realistically, I know you're not. You've probably heard the same thing from your family physician many times before. It hasn't done much good. Fear is not the most effective way to motivate you.

That's too bad. The facts should scare the gluttony out of you. Since obviously it hasn't, all I can hope is that you will become aware of reality and what you are actually doing to yourself.

And decide to change.

If you are obese, some of these problems will overtake you. Guaranteed, or your money back.

One of the best examples I can think of to show you

Composition of Beverages—Alcoholic and Carbonated Nonalcoholic Per 100 Gm![1]

	Food energy (calories)	Protein
Beverages, alcoholic and carbonated non-alcoholic		
Alcoholic		
Beer, alcohol 4.5% by volume (3.6% by weight)	42	.3
Gin, rum, vodka, whisky:		
80-proof (33.4% alcohol by weight)	231	—
86-proof (36.0% alcohol by weight)	249	—
90-proof (37.9% alcohol by weight)	263	—
94-proof (39.7% alcohol by weight)	275	—
100-proof (42.5% alcohol by weight)	295	—
Wines		
Dessert, alcohol 18.8% by volume (15.3% by weight)	137	.1
Table, alcohol 12.2% by volume (9.9% by weight)	85	.1
Carbonated, non-alcoholic		
Carbonated waters:		
sweetened (quinine sodas)	31	—
unsweetened (club sodas)	—	—
Cola type	39	—
Cream sodas	43	—
Fruit-flavored sodas (citrus, cherry, grape, strawberry, Tom Collins mixer, other) (10%-13% sugar)	46	—
Ginger ale, pale dry and golden	31	—
Root beer	41	—
Special dietary drinks with artificial sweetener (less than 1 calorie per ounce)	—	—

[1] From Watt, B. K., and Merrill, A. L.: Composition of foods—raw, processed, prepared, U.S. Department of Agriculture, Agriculture Handbook, No. 8.

how good nutrition can contribute to a longer, healthier life are the people of the Abkhazia region of Soviet Georgia, the same people you see being used by the Dannon Company to promote its product.

Yogurt has very little to do with their long life—often

Carbo-hydrate	Calcium	Phos-phorus	Iron	Thiamine	Ribo-flavin	Niacin
3.8	5	30	Trace	Trace	.03	.6
Trace	—	—	—	—	—	—
Trace	—	—	—	—	—	—
Trace	—	—	—	—	—	—
Trace	—	—	—	—	—	—
Trace	—	—	—	—	—	—
7.7	8	—	—	.01	.02	.2
4.2	9	10	4	Trace	.01	.1
8	—	—	—	—	—	—
—	—	—	—	—	—	—
10	—	—	—	—	—	—
11	—	—	—	—	—	—
12	—	—	—	—	—	—
8	—	—	—	—	—	—
10.5	—	—	—	—	—	—
—	—	—	—	—	—	—

reaching a hundred years or more—or their remarkable energy. It is a combination of many different things, but one of the most important is a good diet.

This diet consists of high-protein, low-fat food with a reduction in total caloric intake. Those with the longest lifespan also avoided cigarettes and liquor, but not wine. Wine, one of them said, contained things that "stimulated the system."

In addition to their diet, the Soviet Georgians also do a great deal of physical work. One of them explained, just prior to his 167th birthday, that he'd been working hard for about *one hundred and fifty years*.

They were also helped by their psychological surroundings, something very hard to categorize but easy to see. They were respected by their families and community and continued to contribute well past the age of what we call retirement. One man who was forced to leave his village began to waste away until he was brought back and became part of the community again.

By any modern standards, the Soviet Georgians lead a simplified life, so it's very hard to translate how they live into terms we can understand and use—except to observe and copy their tradition of physical exercise and good nutrition.

Most dieters either don't know or ignore the fact that their bodies need a minimum amount of nutrients every single day. You have to ingest these nutrients or suffer the consequences. In the mad scramble to lose weight they have self-indulgently put on, many dieters throw out good nutrition.

Throwing out nutrition because you want to lose weight is self-defeating. It makes no sense whatsoever.

Chapter 7

The Two-Legged Machine

Americans love machines. Our preoccupation with them, particularly the automobile, is a thing of legend. To understand good nutrition, think of your body as a machine. If the average American spent as much time and money taking care of his body as he does taking care of his car, we would all be in great shape.

Like a car, your body needs fuel. Cars run on gasoline, your body runs on food. The gasoline in an engine gives it the energy to perform. In your body, food provides energy as well as tissue repair and replacement. If you use the wrong kind of gasoline in your car, the engine will develop carbon deposits and won't run well at all. If you feed your body the wrong kind of food, it won't run well either.

The point of this analogy is this: *Good nutrition means good fuel.*

It should come as no surprise that most people don't equate food with energy. Most people don't really understand what a calorie is.

A calorie isn't a substance even though you might like to think of it as a horrible little creature ruining your life. A calorie is simply a unit of measurement—just like inches and feet—a way of determining the amount of energy or heat produced by the metabolism of the food we eat.

A calorie is a very small amount of energy. A kilocalorie (one thousand calories) is the amount of energy

Daily Energy Requirements*

	Age (yrs.)	Weight (kg.)	Weight (lbs.)	Height (cm.)	Height (ins.)	Calories (kcal.)	Joules (kJ.)
Infants	0.0–0.5	6	14	60	24	kg. × 117	kg. × 489.5
	0.5–1.0	9	20	71	28	kg. × 108	kg. × 451.9
Children	1–3	13	28	86	34	1,300	5,439.2
	4–6	20	44	110	44	1,800	7,531.2
	7–10	30	66	135	54	2,400	10,041.6
Males	11–14	44	97	158	63	2,800	11,715.2
	15–18	61	134	172	69	3,000	12,552.0
	19–22	67	147	172	69	3,000	12,552.0
	23–50	70	154	172	69	2,700	11,296.8
	51+	70	154	172	69	2,400	10,041.6
Females	11–14	44	97	155	62	2,400	10,041.6
	15–18	54	119	162	65	2,100	8,786.4
	19–22	58	128	162	65	2,100	8,786.4
	23–50	58	128	162	65	2,000	8,368.0
	51+	58	128	162	65	1,800	7,531.2
Pregnant						+300	+1,255.2
Lactating						+500	+2,092.0

* Food and Nutrition Board, National Research Council, National Academy of Sciences: Recommended dietary allowances, ed. 8, Washington, D.C., 1974.

it takes to raise one kilogram of water one degree centigrade.

(If you're heavily into the metric system, the units of energy are called joules, named after James Prescott Joule, an English physicist. If you're converting calories to joules, one calorie equals 4.184 joules. Regardless of the fact that nine-tenths of the world uses joules instead of calories, we will continue to use calories in this book.)

The energy equivalents of the three basic forms of food—protein, carbohydrate and fat—are as follows:

One gram of protein yields four calories; one gram of carbohydrate yields four calories; and one gram of fat yields nine calories. Protein is not a primary fuel source but is used in tissue building. Carbohydrates such as sugars and starch are a source of quick energy. Fat, because it is so high in energy potential, is used as a source of stored energy.

The body metabolizes protein into amino acids, carbohydrates into glucose and fats into fatty acids. It is in these three basic forms that food is used by the cells for energy and tissue building.

The body is very fuel-efficient. Unlike an automobile, it doesn't waste anything. What the body doesn't use as energy, it stores as fat. Simple?

Vitamins and minerals, however, should never be confused with our energy needs. They are used to regulate and assist our metabolism, not to run it. We can't live without them, but they don't provide any energy.

Remember that your body's use of energy is constant. Calories are either used or stored every day. They do not pass on to that big calorie counter in the sky. If your body doesn't use them for immediate energy, they end up stuck to your ribs.

Your body needs a great deal of energy just to exist.

Almost two-thirds of the fuel you need is used just keeping you alive without any movement at all—breathing, the beating of your heart, body heat, etc. This is called your *basal metabolism* and it differs from one individual to another. It depends on a number of things—your body size, weight, health, age, sex, etc.

What happens to the other third, the amount of calories left over after your basic metabolic needs are met? That depends on you and you alone. If you lead an active life, if you use a lot of energy, your body will burn up the rest of its caloric intake. If you're like most people, however, you're probably not that active and your body will store the rest of those calories away until a time when you may need them.

When that happens, you're upsetting your energy balance. You're taking in more energy than your body can actively use. So your body does exactly what it's suppose to do, it puts all those extra calories in its reserve tank. *Extra calories are stored as fat!*

Fortunately for us, the human body is the most amazing and most efficient machine known to exist in nature. It is both self-perpetuating and self-repairing. It is also quite capable of self-destruction. It has a great tolerance for chemical and physical abuse—but not indefinitely.

If you cut off the body's supply of oxygen or blood, the effect will be instantaneous—it will die. But if you cut off its supply of vital nutrients—protein, vitamins and minerals—it will suffer for a long time before it tells you that it needs help. If you ignore the danger signals for too long, it will eventually stop running. Permanently.

Good nutrition is the art of supplying the human machine with a proper balance of fuel so that the motor continues to hum along smoothly and adjusts itself to normal variation. Short periods of subnormal nutrition are easily balanced by the body's own self-regulating ability and its own sources of stored nutrients.

It takes time to mess up the human machine. It also takes time to repair it.

Famous Last Words

"I am a yo-yo. I have lost at least five hundred pounds in my life and gained it all back." "You should have seen me last month when I was on the bubblegum and water diet. I lost ten pounds. I really looked good. Now I've gained it all back again." "It must be something in my genes. It's not my fault." "Wait until you see me next month. Then I'll look better."

Chapter 8

The Diet Sweepstakes

Let's take Mrs. Janet Doe of Anywhere, U.S.A. and run her through the first phase of our *Fad Diet Sweepstakes!* This is the part where she gets to choose another one of the exciting new diets on the market. Last year, one of our contestants got to try all seventy-two different diets! This year, who knows? Which one will she pick first? How long will she be able to stick with it? Let's see what's behind the curtain!

Because Janet is trying to get into a new lifestyle, the first one she chooses is: The Zen Macrobiotic Diet! Far out, Janet! For our studio audience and those of you watching breathlessly at home, what Janet is getting here is a delicious ooze of brown rice, soy sauce, cereal and mashed wheat germ all rolled up into one large unappetizing mess. After a few weeks of this diet, Janet is ready to join a religious cult.

In the meantime, Janet may have become anemic and her kidneys may have started to fail. She may also have become emaciated after a few weeks, which is not exactly the same as losing weight. Far out, Janet!

Well, one down and only seventy-one more to go!

The next one Janet chooses is: The Grapefruit Diet! In fact, Janet has so much fruit in her living room that it's beginning to look like an orchard in Orlando. She has grapefruit for breakfast, lunch and dinner. Janet is eating so much grapefruit that her mouth has formed itself into a permanent pucker.

It's too bad that Janet didn't hear what the Post Office Department had to say when it refused to allow the "Super-C Grapefruit Diet Reducing Plan" the right to use the mail.

"The grapefruit itself," they said, "has no special properties as a metabolizer of fat . . . [and] it could be harmful to persons with certain kinds of heart or kidney problems." Janet is off the grapefruit diet now, but she still harbors a certain resentment against citrus fruit. Last week in the supermarket, she tried to strangle a bag of grapefruit to death.

For her next choice, Janet has decided on one of our old favorites: The-Count-Your-Calories-Every-Single-Time-You-Eat-Diet! This diet is favored by people who own stock in electronic calculator companies, because that's what it takes to find out what you're having for dinner. After a couple weeks of patiently assembling a list of the foods she can eat, then weighing in every single portion, then struggling with hunger pangs be-tween meals, Janet is ready to rip things out of the walls.

There are, Janet finds, problems with this diet that she actually hadn't anticipated. It takes forever. Janet is losing her mind but not much weight.

Meanwhile, Janet is beginning to feel like a stock character in "I Love Lucy" what with her calorie charts, her scales and her list of calorie "don'ts" a mile and a half long. Her kitchen looks like a free fire zone. She quickly loses patience with the diet, but not much weight.

Well, back to square one for Janet!

Janet stumbles on to the next one: The-Low-Or-No-Carbohydrate-Diet! This one and all its variations is nothing new, Janet learns.

What Janet also learns is that she has to keep her measuring spoons handy for this diet, too. She has to learn how to keep her carbohydrate intake—and she's never really too sure just what's a carbohydrate and what isn't—between thirty and fifty grams a day. This is metric, right? And very tricky, too. Through trial and a lot of error, she figures out that if she consumes even a few grams above the mark, she won't lose very much weight.

Janet tries every conceivable variation of this diet. First, there's the Air Force Diet which has nothing to do with the U.S. Air Force. Then there's the Drinking Man's Diet—if he can do it, so can she!—which not only adds empty calories to her diet but also increases the amount of saturated fat in her blood stream and may eventually increase her chances of a heart attack.

Well, let's let Janet rest for awhile, because by this time she really needs it. She's been diet-hyped right out of shape. She's disappointed, demoralized and depressed. She hasn't lost any weight, either.

If we wanted to, we could run our mythical Janet through fad diets for the rest of the century. We could, for instance, put her on the high protein, free fat diet advocated by Dr. Robert Atkins.

On Atkins' diet, she may lose some weight, but whether she loses weight or not on this diet, it will not help her keep her weight under control once she's lost it. It requires another cavalry charge of food lists, calorie counters and a perpetual calendar for scheduling.

There's also the high protein, massive water diet of Dr. Irwin Maxwell Stillman. His gimmick was the eighty ounces of water you were suppose to drink every day. The water in Stillman's diet doesn't do anything at all. She drinks it and it gets passed right out. It doesn't take any weight with it, but it certainly keeps her kidneys flushed.

Stillman's diet is also boring. Eating one kind of food constantly will drive Janet crazy after a week and that will give her ample encouragement to cheat.

The Diet Sweepstakes could continue with these other fad diets: The Ten Day-Ten Pounds Off Menu, the Nibbling Diet, the Rice Diet, the Hot Dog Diet, the Vegetable and Fruit Diet, the Milk Diet, the Milk and Bananas Diet, the Buttermilk and Cottage Cheese Diet, the Strawberry and Cream Diet, The Meat and Mushroom Diet, the Egg and Yogurt Diet, the Egg and Wine Diet, the Egg and Orange Diet, and on and on, ad nauseam.

Then, of course, thre's the one they call The Ultimate Diet—Total Starvation!

Total Insanity!

The Protein Sparing Modified Fast (PSMF) is the current diet fad in this country. Those who use it call it the ultimate way to lose weight. Why not? You give up eating completely and replace it with a predigested liquid protein. Except for some vitamins and minerals, this is your sole source of nutrition. In recent months, some specialists have changed to edible protein sources in place of the liquid form. (This emphasizes my principles about the need for eating.)

Obviously you will lose weight rapidly on the PSMF.

The number of calories you're consuming each day is fewer than five hundred. That's not the problem.

This technique was designed for the morbidly obese, not for the average person who wants to lose less than thirty pounds. The PSMF is also unnatural, extremely severe, and should be carried out only in a hospital under strict medical supervision. This is how it was originally designed. It is not a "do it yourself" game.

But the PSMF fails where it counts the most. It takes the weight off, but makes only a superficial pass at changing your eating habits. Once the crashing ends, the person who had bad eating habits starts eating again. Nothing has changed. The new thin person thinks and eats like the old fat person.

Your body has been put under considerable stress. You have sacrificed and, in effect, starved yourself. The rewards are fleeting. Out goes the liquid protein and in comes the new river of calories.

Chapter 9

Mother's Little Helpers

The amount of money Americans spend on diets and dieting has been estimated at anywhere from a half-billion to ten billion dollars per year. The money goes for everything over, under and around the counter. There are pills, creams, lotions, tonics, books, pamphlets, machines, exercisers, psychiatrists, clubs, therapies, clinics, surgery, charts, lists, diet foods, diet drinks, hypnosis, and even a machine that will yell at you each time you open your refrigerator door.

What usually happens to people that buy these treatments is depressing. The vast majority will gain back every single pound they lose, probably within the first six months. When people talk about criminals who can't stay out of jail, they talk about repeaters. It's the same thing with dieters and fad diets. They almost always go back to jail. They do not pass "Go" or collect $200 either.

Most, if not all, of these diet treatments fail to take into consideration what is most important for long-term weight control—the re-education of the dieter. There's no sense in losing weight if you're going to get it back a year later. A knowledge of nutrition, exercise and self-control are essential.

You must develop a *new food lifestyle*.

Let's take another look at some of these other approaches to weight loss so you can understand why they don't work.

Pills

It was called Bel-Doxin when it was taken off the market a few years ago. Like many of the "diet" pills that are advertised in the back of magazines, it promised to suppress the appetite and help you lose all the fat you wanted. At the same time, it promised you could still eat as much as you wanted. Their advertising made Bel-Doxin sound like the greatest thing since night baseball. Like the Anapax Diet Plan Tablets in 1970, which were also taken off the market by the New York Attorney General, Bel-Doxin appealed to the millions of dieters who wanted the magic of a pill.

Bel-Doxin, unfortunately, contained the drug scopolamine aminoxide, which made the taker drowsy, and, so the manufacturer apparently figured, too tired to eat. The manufacturer also failed to tell anybody that prolonged use of the drug—particularly by someone who was unknowingly allergic to it—could cause serious side effects, such as falling asleep at the wheel of your car while driving under its influence.

There are other forms of "diet" pills, the kind prescribed by many physicians. They are amphetamines, but they go by a lot of other names, too. Often they are called anti-depressants because they give the user a feeling of well-being. When you take amphetamines (speed, uppers, crystal, meth, etc.) you feel like King Kong. You talk a lot. Sometimes you just babble incoherently. You have more energy then you ever thought possible. Sleep? Who needs sleep? When you leap out of bed in the morning you feel like a 747 at full throttle.

The pills are supposed to cut your appetite, and for a while, they do just that. Eventually, however, that effect wears off. Then you begin to feel just a little bit edgey. Loud noises begin to bother you. You start to yell at people a lot. If you smoke cigarettes, you smoke them in a chain, often lighting a new one before crushing the old one out. You find you're becoming *very* nervous.

Finally, you begin to think that people are picking on you. Why are all these people whispering about you when your back is turned? Your whole life is turning into a series of incredible highs and excruciating lows.

Congratulations, you are now a speed freak. Or, as some psychiatrists put it, a paranoid schizophrenic.

If this isn't bad enough, you still haven't learned how to control your eating habits. When you finally get off the drug—withdrawl from speed is remarkably unpleasant—you find you still eat like a horse. You may never have stopped eating like one at all. You still eat junk food. If you were on the drug long enough, you may have done permanent damage to your mind and body.

Pills of any sort are a shaky and dangerous proposition, despite the fact that taking them is easy. You do nothing but put it in your mouth. What a pill won't do is very plain. It will not help you control your weight in the long run. Nor will it protect your health the way natural food will!

The Machines

Reducing machines are predicated upon the strange notion that unlimited exercise will translate into unlimited weight loss. In theory this is true but in reality it is very difficult to achieve. For the grossly overweight person it is, for all practical purposes, impossible. But millions of people have bought these exercise products believing these outrageous claims.

Exercise *can* contribute to weight control and well-being, but only as part of an *overall program*, not as a single cure-all. Exercise does a number of good things. It can firm up your muscles, it can help your heart and your lungs, improve your circulation, and you may look and feel better because of it. But unless you're prepared to spend three-quarters of your time in a gym, exercise *alone* won't make you lose weight.

The Tone-O-Matic was a machine that promised to "whittle inches off your waist," but most of the "whittling" was confined to people's pockets. The Federal Trade Commission (FTC) took an active dislike to Tone-O-Matic's chiseling and said the machine wouldn't do anything except injure a few people who wore the weighted belt around the house.

The government, however, was about four months too late in scolding Tone-O-Matic. It had all ready gone out of business when the FTC issued their warning, leaving a string of unhappy and unsatisfied customers in its wake.

The Relaxacizor—another great name—managed to gross forty million dollars in twenty-one years of business before the government closed down the plant because the Relaxacizor was not only a fraud but also deadly. It consisted of another belt, but this one passed an electrical current around the abdomen of the wearer. This, said the manufacturer, would firm up the tummy. A Federal court thought it might do that to somebody permanently. Among its other wonderful properties, the court said, was the possibility it could cause heart failure.

They come in all sizes and prices, these machines and devices. The Sauna Belt, a plastic, inflatable belt that let your stomach area "steam" during exercise, sold quite well—six hundred thousand units at ten dollars a piece. Since it was sold through the mail, the Post Office intervened on behalf of the fourteen thousand people who demanded refunds.

On and on they go in a continuous line, bringing money to the manufacturers and disappointment to the customer. Avoid them completely. They don't do anything, they cost a great deal of money and, ultimately, they leave you feeling more hopeless than ever.

Because they don't do what they claim.

So the question remains: Is there a weight control method that is both safe and effective and won't drive you crazy?

The answer to that is yes.

These other methods are fads, and chances are you'll gain back all the weight you may have lost. They do not take into account good nutrition or good eating habits. They may endanger your physical and mental health. Crash diets are just plain bad for you.

Remember, airplanes crash, people do not.

Chapter 10

Who's Fat? I'm Just a Little Plump!

One is overweight who weighs between ten and twenty percent more than what his or her ideal weight should be. What is ideal weight? The only reasonable guide we have are the insurance company height and weight tables. The term overweight is something that can't be defined specifically, but you probably know it if you are. An obese person is obviously overweight, but an overweight person is not necessarily obese.

There are exceptions. For instance, a professional athlete might easily fall into the plus-ten-percent weight category. That extra weight on the athlete is muscle, not fat, and that makes all the difference. The athlete in this case is not really overweight; he's just big.

Another example. A man who stands 6′ 4″ tall and weighs 225 pounds may be overweight. According to the tables, a man that tall with a large frame should weigh somewhere between 182 and 204. But many nutritionists add approximately ten percent to any given weight as a safe range. So our man may not be overweight.

The very best definition of overweight is the one you set for yourself with the advice of your own doctor.

If you don't like the way you look, then you may very well be overweight. However, your doctor may simply suggest some additional exercise and some muscle toning to solve the problem. This is particularly true of men who have trouble seeing their shoes because of a bulging middle. It may be that they are overweight; it may also be a simple case of sagging muscles.

A person who has been fairly slim all his life may wake up in middle age to find he's developed a pot belly. Middle age is the most difficult time for weight control. You become less active during these years and your life style—both in and out of work—is likely to become more sedentary. The problem here is that you're still eating the same amount of food as you did when you were younger, but you're not doing enough to burn it up.

Soon you may find yourself exceeding the ten percent weight gain range. If this happens, then you are not overweight—you are obese!

Obesity means grossly overweight. Anyone who carries twenty percent more than what his or her normal weight should be, is obese. You know when you're obese because life becomes an extended misery. You could become short of breath. You can't wear the clothes you bought not too long ago.

You are often as wide as the sidewalk.

At least thirty percent of all overweight Americans could be classified as obese. Thirty percent! What is as important is what obesity can do to you. It can foul you up so badly that you may become a diabetic. It can promote diseases of the digestive system such as ulcers, diabetes and colitis. It can give you a stroke or cause hypertension. It can give you severe arthritis or destroy your heart. It can kill.

Obesity does kill!

That horrifying litany is the inevitable result of obesity. In the meantime, you have to contend with the psychological problems. According to one researcher, obese adolescents, particularly girls, showed the same type of mental symptoms recognized by psychologists in severely oppressed minorities: paranoia, passivity and withdrawal.

Obesity can be the result of many factors except one: heredity. There is nothing genetic about obesity. If you are obese, however, your children stand a good chance of becoming obese themselves. In other words, obesity can be *learned*.

Obesity can also be the result of social factors, such as income and eating patterns. Early overfeeding of school children can contribute to a pattern of obesity in later life. It may also be caused by an unresolved emotional problem. People often over-eat to compensate for something else—loneliness, boredom, anxiety or repressed anger.

If you are obese, your doctor has probably warned and scolded you a hundred times, and it hasn't helped very much. What your doctor is waiting for is a change in your attitude. You may listen to him after your first heart attack or your first stroke.

You may also be dead.

Treating the overweight person is difficult, but the treatment of obesity is much more complex. It can be anything from keeping extensive records of what you eat to planned interruptions of the eating process itself. It may go so far as the costly and dangerous practice of surgically removing a large portion of your intestine.

The best way to understand the difference between obesity and overweight is this: Being overweight is uncomfortable. Being obese is lethal.

Chapter 11
The Basics: Fat

Here are a few non-fattening facts for you to chew over. Americans eat too much fat. Almost half—forty percent —of our total calories comes from fat. The average person eats *one hundred* pounds of fat a year, but *needs* less than twenty-five.

Fat is a highly concentrated form of energy. It has twice the energy potential of carbohydrates and protein. Carbohydrates, however, are more easily digested than fats and are a source of quick energy. Fats are a source of stored energy. The body stores the lipids—the scientists' word for what we call fat—in the cells which are created specifically for that purpose—adipose cells.

Fat, in all its forms, is what's making you overweight.

This is how it works. During digestion, the body breaks down the fats you eat into three basic substances: glycerol, steroids and fatty acids.

Glycerol is a water-soluble form of fat, which means it can travel through the bloodstream easily because blood, if you didn't know, is water-based. (If necessary, glycerol can be used to form glucose.)

The only steroid you really must know about is cholesterol. Cholesterol is a thick white substance that is fat-related and synthesized in the liver. Even if you ate nothing that contained cholesterol, your body would still manufacture about two grams of it a day.

Unfortunately, Americans eat many things that contain cholesterol, and this increases the amount of it that is synthesized by the liver. An easy guide to cholesterol is that plants and plant food contain no cholesterol. Animal food—like eggs, liver, milk, and cheese—contains cholesterol.

If you take in too much cholesterol, you simply accelerate the process of atherosclerosis (hardening of the arteries). Cholesterol may also build up in the gall bladder and form gall stones. A certain amount of cholesterol is necessary to keep the body functioning—it is used by the brain and liver and can be changed into vitamin D when the skin is exposed to the ultraviolet rays of the sun. But, by and large, Americans eat too much food containing cholesterol and that is not good for anybody.

The third basic fat substances are the fatty acids, *the* refined fuel unit of fat that the body uses as energy. The two types of fatty acids are saturated and unsaturated. Anyone who has seen a margarine ad on television knows about saturated and unsaturated fats.

Saturated fats are animal in origin, and because they are fairly solid, they are more difficult for the body to break down. They also contribute to atherosclerosis. Unsaturated fats are plant fats—oils made from olives, peanuts, corn and safflower—and their use helps lower the amount of cholesterol in the blood.

(Remember, there is no caloric difference between butter and margarine. They have the same number of calories but margarine contains more unsaturated fats than butter and that's why doctors recommend its use.)

Once the body has broken down the fat into fatty acids, they are burned as fuel within the cells. Unfortunately, since most people eat too much fat, these excess fatty acids undergo another change. They are changed *back* into tissue fat and stored in the adipose cells for future use. In the case of the chronically overweight, "future use" rarely, if ever, arrives and the fat stays put.

There have been a number of studies concerning the nature of the adipose cells in the body. Some people, particularly those who were overfed during infancy and early childhood, may actually develop more adipose cells than necessary, accelerating their tendency towards obesity. While none of this is conclusive, the studies point towards the idea that early nutrition helps determine your fat capacity later on. The culprit in both cases is nutritional misadventure during the formative years. Once someone reaches adulthood, the number of adipose cells remains the same.

What happens during a period of weight loss is also being investigated. Findings indicate that the size of the adipose cells decreases, but that their number remains the same. If your weight gain began as a child or during adolescence, it means you will always have more of a weight problem than someone who gained excess weight later in life.

Chapter 12

Carbohydrates

Carbohydrates, like fat, provide the body with energy. Unlike fat, however, carbohydrates are the body's main source of quick energy because the digestive system is able to break them down rapidly and pass them along to the cells. If the body is confronted with an excess of carbohydrate—just like excess fat—it is changed into tissue fat and stored in the adipose cells.

There are basically three different kinds of carbohydrates: monosaccharides, disaccharides and polysaccharides.

The simplest form of carbohydrate is the monosaccharide or simple sugar. Glucose is the most common monosaccharide. It is also what the body uses as fuel. During digestion, all carbohydrates are broken down into glucose and glycogen. (Glycogen is not used as a fuel but is stored in very small amounts in the liver and muscles and, like stored fat, is kept in reserve in case of an emergency.)

Fructose, also a monosaccharide, is found in fruits and honey. Fructose is the main reason you don't have to sweeten fruit juice. Nature has already sweetened it for you, making it an easy source of weight gain.

Disaccharides, as the prefix "di" might suggest, are slightly more complex than monosaccharides. Sucrose— common refined white sugar—is a disaccharide. So is lactose, the sugar in milk.

Polysaccharides are complex carbohydrates. They include starches, cellulose (fiber) and glycogen. Glycogen is made from glucose. The others are usually found growing out of the ground.

As I said before, you've been eating too many simple carbohydrates—specifically sugar—and not enough complex ones. This change in diet has helped make us a nation of malnourished fat people.

Simple carbohydrates do very little for you except provide a quick source of energy. At one time, starches were the main source of carbohydrates and gave people vitamins, minerals and fiber along with with quick energy. Sucrose gives you what a lot of people call "empty" calories. Most of the evils in your current diet can be traced to this increased consumption of sugar.

Some researchers go one step further and question whether we need carbohydrates in our diet at all. Donald S. McLaren, a nutritionist and author of *Nutrition and Its Disorders*, says, "There is no evidence to suggest that carbohydrate is an essential part of the human diet. The energy it provides can be obtained from other sources. Health was maintained by Arctic explorers on a purely meat diet and many meat-eating tribes have habitually very little carbohydrate in their diet."

If your consumption of sugar has reached the point of wretched excess, this might be a solution to keep in mind. At the very least, it means that lowering the amount of carbohydrate you take in is a good idea.

Chapter 13
Protein

Protein, either animal or vegetable, is what the body needs for tissue building. It is the basis of all cell structure and the primary component of all body tissue. Sufficient protein cannot be stored in the body like fat and must be replenished every day.

As a general rule, protein provides very little of the body's energy needs. In some emergency or starvation instances, however, protein can be changed to provide *almost all* of the body's energy needs, but on a day-to-day basis this is not the case.

Protein is a Greek word meaning "primary" and was first used by a Dutch chemist who knew very little about it but was apparently blessed with some sort of prescience. When protein is digested and broken down by the body, it reveals its essential ingredients: amino acids, the basis of life. (At one time, when it was first formed, the world was literally covered with an amino acid ocean.)

There are, in all, 22 amino acids. They must be present in certain amounts and combinations for different tissues throughout the body. Of the 22, there are eight essential amino acids that the body *must* have to function correctly, They are, in no particular order: Leucine, Isoleucine, Valine, Lysine, Methionine, Phenylalanine, Threonine and Tryptophane. (Together they sound a little like the cast of a Greek tragedy.) These eight essential amino acids must be present in the body *at the same time* and in certain specific proportions in order to be effective. If they aren't, the body can't use them.

The quality of a protein source is judged solely on the presence of these eight essential amino acids plus variables of the others. If not all are present, then that source is considered of low nutrient value. There are only a limited number of foods that deliver the right amount of amino acids—eggs, milk, cheese, meat, fish and poultry.

The average man needs approximately fifty-six grams of protein every day. The average woman needs forty-six grams of protein every day. That means that *everybody* has to have between five and six ounces of protein daily and that amount *must* provide those eight essential amino acids to protect and rebuild the body's tissue.

There is an amino acid pool in the liver that maintains a small storage supply of these amino acids of the body and it must be re-supplied regularly. This pool also takes care of your body's protein needs between meals and during sleep (when not feeding).

If you suddenly stopped supplying your body with protein, your amino acid pool would eventually be depleted and the process of tissue building would stop. Eventually, much of the muscle and organ tissue would be used for energy. By maintaining a steady supply of protein—and by keeping your intake of carbohydrates and fats low—you're saving the lean tissue so that the *stored fat* can be used as energy.

This is particularly important for dieters. During a

period of weight loss, protein needs are often neglected and the dieter suffers. But whether you're dieting or not, the body must have protein because any kind of growth needs protein. Your hair and nails—almost one hundred percent protein—are growing, your skin is constantly replacing itself and your blood cells change completely every four months.

It has been argued by some nutritionists that Americans eat too much protein, since such a large portion of our national diet consists of meat (three-fifths of our protein comes from animal sources). What is troubling about our consumption of meat is not that it is high in protein but that it is also high in saturated fats.

The more red meat we eat, the more saturated fats we take in, and that contributes both to high cholesterol and the increased possibility of heart attack. It also contributes to our weight problem. Vegetarians often have less trouble with both these problems because of the source of their protein—things like soybeans, chick peas and nuts. Plant protein is high in unsaturated fats.

Another problem with getting your protein from animal sources is money. Meat costs a lot these days. You might consider, if you're so inclined, increasing the amount of plant protein in your diet. You would be saving money *and* cutting down dramatically on the amount of saturated fat.

The most important thing to remember about protein and all those amino acids is that you need them every day and you need them in the right quantities. If any one of them is missing in your diet, the process of tissues building and protection will not happen.

In the final analysis, protein is the single most important thing you need for good health. Next to oxygen, of course.

Chapter 14
Vitamins/Minerals

Vitamins and minerals are essential to good nutrition. As with protein, you cannot live without either one. They have to be taken everyday in certain amounts, or deficiencies will develop. They are needed in much smaller amounts, however, than the other nutrients.

Vitamins have certain characteristics: They cannot be manufactured by the body and most cannot be stored there, either. Some are water-soluble while others work only with fatty acids.

The study of vitamins is relatively new and research has been confined to this century. The word vitamin was coined by a Polish chemist with the unusual name of Casimir Funk who experimented with pigeons in London in the early 1900s. After changing the birds' diet, he discovered they soon developed paraylsis. In the process of finding out why, Funk named the missing substance vitamine—"being vital to life." Eventually the "e" was dropped and the word ended up as "vitamin."

Vitamin deficiencies were once the scourge of the world and we have all heard the stories about the British Navy and scurvy. (James Lind, a British surgeon, decided that what the sailors needed was an ounce of lemon or lime juice every day to combat scurvy. This is why the English were called Limies.) Other vitamin deficiency diseases such as rickets, pellagra and beriberi have also been the subject of much legend and lore.

The fact is that there are at least thirteen essential vitamins that you must have every day of your life though the amounts are often ridiculously small. For instance, you need approximately two micrograms of Cobalamin (B_{12}) every day or you may develop pernicious anemia.

Vitamins do not provide energy or make you lose or gain weight. They are, practically speaking, the body's supervisors and assistants. Their presence allows the other nutrients—protein, carbohydrates and fats—to do their stuff as normally as possible. The result is a balanced normal metabolism.

Some vitamins help control specific body functions. Vitamin A, for example, helps the eye to adapt to changes in light. Vitamin A deficiency can cause night blindness.

Minerals also help supervise the body's metabolism. Without minerals (and vitamins) we would all be in a state of nutritional chaos. Minerals, however, are generally found in the body in much larger quantities than vitamins. (Those minerals required in large amounts are called major minerals; those required in smaller amounts are called trace elements.)

Calcium—a major mineral—is almost two percent of our body weight and the average adult has about three pounds of calcium, mostly in the bones, in his or her body. You need about one gram of calcium a day to maintain proper nutrition.

On the other hand, the amount of iodine needed every day is incredibly small—about twenty-five micrograms.

Iodine is stored in the thyroid gland and helps synthesize the thyroid hormone, which in turn helps regulate the body's metabolism. You get iodine mostly from salt.

The point of all this is simple: Whether you need one gram or twenty-five micrograms, you have to maintain *all* of these essential minerals all the time. A lack of any one of them can cause problems. Some studies show that an iron deficiency is an all too common occurrence in the American diet. And a deficiency of either vitamins or minerals doesn't necessarily show itself right away—not until it creates an illness.

This is particularly true during dieting, when even a minor deficiency may cause serious problems. That's why an understanding of good nutrition is so important when you diet.

The role of these nutrients can't be overstated. Without them, you simply wouldn't be able to use the food you eat.

There have been a number of studies linking certain vitamin and mineral deficiencies with mental illnesses such as depression and schizophrenia. Future research may prove that there is an even wider range of illnesses, both mental and physical, linked to vitamin and mineral deficiencies.

Vitamin and Mineral Sources

VITAMINS

A	Fish-liver oils, liver, butter, cream, milk, cheese, egg yolk, dark green and yellow vegetables, yellow fruits, and fortified margarine.
D	Fish-liver oils, fortified milk, exposure to sunlight; very small amounts in butter, liver, and egg yolks.
E	Oils of wheat germ, rice germ, germs of seds; greeen leafy vegetables, nuts, and legumes.
Niacin	Lean meat, liver, kidney, wholegrain and enriched cereals and breads, green vegetables, peanuts, yeast.
B_6 (Pyridoxine)	Wheat germ, meat, liver, kidney, Whole-grain and enriched cereals and breads, green vegetables, peanuts, yeast.
B_{12}	Milk, eggs, cheese, liver, kidney, meats contain small amounts.
Biotin	Liver, kidney, molasses, milk, yeast, egg yolk, and green vegetables.
C	Citrus fruits, strawberries, cantaloupe, tomatoes, cabbage, potatoes, green peppers, and broccoli.
Folic Acid	Green leafy vegetables, liver, kidney, yeast.

B₁ (Thiamine)	Pork, liver, heart, kidney, mlik, yeast, whole-grain and enriched cereals and breads, soybeans, legumes, peanuts, and wheat germ.
B₂ (Riboflavin)	Milk, powdered whey, liver, kidney, heart, meats, eggs, green leafy vegetables, dried yeast.
Pantothenic Acid	Almost universally present in plant and animal tissue. Loss of 50% in milling of flour; 33% lost in cooking meat.
K	Green leafy vegetables such as alfalfa, spinach, cabbage; liver.

MINERALS

Calcium	Milk, hard cheese, and in kale, mustard, turnip and collard greens. Also some in oysters, shrimp, salmon, clams, and in other dairy products.
Phosphorous	Milk, cheese, egg yolk, meat, fish, fowl, legumes, nuts, whole-grain cereals.
Iodine	Iodized salt best source; also salt water fish.
Iron	Liver, meat, egg yolk, legumes, molasses, dark green leafy vegetables, peaches, prunes, apricots, raisins, enriched flour and cereal.
Fluoride	Milk, eggs, and fish; many communities add fluorine to drinking water.

| Potassium | Meat, fish, fowl, cereals, fruits, vegetables. |

| Chlorine
Copper
Zinc
Manganese
Sulfur
Cobalt
Molybdenum | Trace elements found in green and yellow vegetables. |

Nutrients And What They Do

This section will show you what the various nutrients do in your system. With this list, you can also check to see if you are suffering from a deficiency of any one of them.

VITAMINS	*FUNCTION*
A	Necessary for cell growth and the repair of tissue. Helps maintain healthy eyes, skin, gums and teeth. Also fights infection. A vitamin A deficiency may result in night blindness, dry skin, fatigue and an increased susceptibility to infection. (Overdose possible with excessive amount—not common.)
D	Essential for bones and teeth. Vitamin D helps the body absorb and use calcium and phosphorus. Also helps stabilize the nervous system. A defici-

VITAMINS   FUNCTION

	ency may result in poor bone and teeth formation.
E	Vitamin E protects certain fat-soluble vitamins, increases the life span of red blood cells and prevents blood clots. A deficiency may result in the destruction of red blood cells and the deterioration of the muscles. Deficiency not common in humans.
Niacin	Helps the body metabolize carbohydrates. Protects the skin, tongue, nervous and digestive systems. A deficiency results in pellagra, which may cause depression, diarrhea and skin disease.
B_6 (Pyridoxine)	Essential for protein metabolism and helps in the formation of the iron in red blood cells. A deficiency causes irritability, nervousness, dizziness, and nausea. Women who take birth control pills may need more of this vitamin than others.
B_{12}	Essential for the formation of red blood cells and to maintain a healthy nervous system. A deficiency causes pernicious anemia; in children a deficiency may result in retarded growth.

VITAMINS	FUNCTION

Biotin — Helps the body use the other B vitamins as well as helping to metabolize protein, fat and carbohydrate. Depression, skin trouble and muscle pain may result from a deficiency of Biotin, although it is uncommon with a normal diet.

C — Helps heal wounds, and increases the body's resistance to infection. It also keeps blood vessels strong and improves tissue repair. A deficiency may result in bleeding gums, slow-healing wounds and excessive bruising.

Folic acid — Folic acid is essential for the creation of red blood cells. It also helps metabolize proteins. If you are deficient in Folic acid you may become anemic and suffer from intestinal problems. Folic acid works closely with B_{12}.

Thiamine (B_1) — Helps metabolize carbohydrates and also aids normal appetite and strenthens the nerve tissue. Problems resulting from a Thiamine deficiency are: heart trouble, loss of appetite, fatigue and nerve disorders such as depression.

Riboflavin (B_2) — Helps metabolize carbohydrate and

VITAMINS   FUNCTION

protein by enzyme action. It also
builds antibodies and red blood cells.
A Riboflavin deficiency could result
in lip sores and cracks, retarded
growth and skin problems.

Pantothenic acid   Helps to control the blood sugar
level as a coenzyme in carbohydrate
and fat metabolism. It also helps to
utilize other vitamins and hormones.
Without Pantothenic acid you may
be overly susceptible to disease, but
a deficiency is rare, since it is available in most foods.

MINERALS   FUNCTION

Calcium   Essential for strong bones and teeth.
(99 percent is in bones and teeth.)
Also helps the muscles, nerves and
heart. Involved in blood coagulation.
A calcium deficiency may cause brit-
tle bones, bad teeth, and nerve damage. Absorption is difficult and frequently below normal.

Phosphorus   Helps your body use calcium for
bones and teeth. Also helps in the
metabolism of food. Phosphorus has
more functions than any other mineral. A deficiency causes the same
problems as calcium.

MINERALS   FUNCTION

Iodine

Iodine promotes growth and helps regulate the body's production of energy. It is essential to the proper function of the thyroid gland.

Iron

Iron helps carry oxygen to the cells and is essential for the formation of hemoglobin. It also aids the metabolism of protein. Constipation, anemia, and general lack of energy result from an iron deficiency.

Magnesium

Magnesium joins with some enzymes to help the body metabolize fat, protein, carbohydrate, phosphorus and calcium. A magnesium deficiency may cause nervousness and tremors. (Sixty percent is found in bones and teeth.)

Copper

Helps form red blood cells and aids in the release of iron to form hemoglobin. A deficiency may cause weakness and skin sores. (A trace element.)

Zinc

Helps heal wounds and aids in the metabolism of phosphorus. Zinc is also found in the male reproductive system. A lack of zinc may cause retarded growth and a delayed sexual

MINERALS   FUNCTION

maturity. Zinc also helps in the production of insulin.

Fluoride

Helps eliminate tooth decay in children. (A trace element.)

Potassium

Essential along with calcium for nervous impulses and muscular function—especially in the heart. Takes part in the formation of protein and glycogen. Essential for acid-base and fluid balance, along with sodium. Stored and functions mainly inside the cells. Excretion guarded by the kidneys. A healthy kidney means proper balance of potassium in the body. The body needs 2–6 grams a day.

Water

Although not really a mineral or vitamin, water is the vehicle for an metabolic processes. It is essential for life.

Chapter 15

Fiber: I Knew Him When They Called Him "Bulk"

How does fiber, or bulk, affect the diet? First we have to know exactly what fiber is. Fiber is the undigestible part of food, specifically plant food. It includes things like cellulose, or the walls surrounding the plant cells. Plants like celery, asparagus, corn, beans and broccoli are high in fiber. So are foods like whole wheat bread, bran cereals and raw fruit.

What does it do? The main job of fiber, or bulk, is to help maintain normal bowel movements. (There is no rule about "normal regularity." Everybody has his own rhythm. For some people it's daily. For others, it's twice a week.)

Unfortunately, with all the processed food we eat today, we don't get very much bulk in our diet. When you start on a weight loss program, the amount of bulk is decreased again. With a combination like this, it's no wonder that our pattern of regular bowel movements is disrupted.

There is another benefit of fiber that is directly related to weight control. High-fiber foods are high in carbohydrates, but the body doesn't use all the calories in these foods simply because it doesn't use the fiber. Those calories in the fiber are passed out of the body.

This lack of fiber in our diet is fairly new. As food processing became more commonplace, the amount of fiber in our food decreased. This is especially true of bread. At one time all bread was made from whole wheat —they used the whole grain including the wheat germ and the outer wall of bran. Wheat germ is high in vitamins. That's why most white breads (and flour) have to be fortified with vitamins. They not only took out the fiber, they also took out *all of the natural vitamins*, as well. This is called progress.

Can increasing the amount of fiber in your diet help you lose weight? Yes, if by increasing the amount of fiber, you also begin to decrease the amount of refined food that you eat. However if you continue to gobble junk food and have one or two bowls of bran flakes every day, you will not lose weight. You may become as regular as the sunrise but you won't lose any weight.

Both our government, in the form of the Senate Select Committee on Nutrition and Human Needs, and the Canadian government have recommended an increased amount of fiber in the diet. They suggest more raw vegetables, whole grained breads and dried beans, such as lentils. At the same time, they also recommend decreasing the amount of sugar consumed by fifty percent and the amount of fat by at least twenty-five percent. These recommendations must go together to have any impact on your problem.

There are also indications that fiber aids digestion and that it may contribute to the prevention of ailments such as ulcers, tooth decay and cancer of the colon. The thinking seems to be that because fiber passes through the system quickly, it reduces the amount of carcinogens (suspected cancer-producing substances found in some processed foods today) in the digestive tract. A number of researchers say we should increase the amount of fiber in our diets by ten to fifteen grams per day.

Many people are moving away from overly refined foods towards what has been called a more natural diet. It is natural in the sense that before the onslaught of processed food this is what everyone ate—more fiber, more complex carbohydrates and much less sugar.

If eating more fiber and more fiber-containing foods would lead to a decreased consumption of sugar and refined foods—whose major ingredient is sugar—that in itself would be reason enough for you to consider it.

Chapter 16
The Role of Insulin

In an earlier chapter I told you how the body uses carbohydrates to produce glucose, the body's major fuel. After digestion changes the carbohydrates into glucose, it is then passed through the blood stream to the cells. This is the *blood sugar*, and the controlling agent of blood sugar is insulin. Insulin is the hormone produced in the pancreas, and it does a number of interesting things.

1. It helps increase the permeability of the cell wall, to make it easier for the glucose to get into the cell and be burned for energy.

2. It helps convert glucose to glycogen. Glycogen is then stored in small amounts in the liver and muscle tissue.

3. The most important function of insulin in overweight and obese people: *Insulin increases the conversion of glucose to fat for storage.*

How does this affect you? In a normal metabolism, insulin controls the levels of blood sugar. As with every other process in the body, there is a normal range for these levels. If the body fails to produce a sufficient amount of insulin to control the blood sugar, you are a diabetic. If insulin is overproduced and your blood sugar level is too low, then you may have hypoglycemia.

There is a direct link between excess weight and diabetes, because the body's natural insulin/blood sugar level balance is severely upset. Because you eat too much, the pancreas has to work overtime to produce enough insulin to cope with the excess blood sugar. After that, the insulin does what it's supposed to do by accelerating the conversion of all that extra glucose to fat so that it can be stored in the adipose cells. That's right, you get fat—or fatter! This is a vicious cycle and one that has to be controlled at the source—your mouth.

A normal blood sugar level (which may range anywhere from 70 to 120 milligrams of glucose per 100 milliliters of blood) will make you feel relativey energetic and vital. Your body will be getting the correct amount of fuel and you feel good. Once your blood sugar level starts to fall, however, fatigue may set in. If you are a chronic overeater, your blood sugar levels have been abnormally high and you must keep them at that level to feel energetic.

In other words, you have to *eat more than most people to feel good.* Your body is so out of balance that it doesn't respond to lower sugar levels, even though those levels are well within the normal range.

As you start to decrease the amount of food you eat—and your blood sugar level—you probably won't feel as good as you did when you were busy stuffing yourself. This is to be expected and is only temporary. Your body is readjusting itself to the change. Eventually it will become accustomed to a lower blood sugar level and a lower production of insulin. When that happens, your "energy" will return.

At the same time, you will develop a feeling of well-being by eating less!

"Permanent weight loss can only be effected by a change in life style"

> Cathy Kapica Cyborski
> AMA Dept. of Foods & Nutrition
> Chicago

Chapter 17
Before the Diet

I'd like you to eavesdrop on a typical lecture that I used to give some of my pregnant patients:

"Joanne," I'd start out, "you're gaining too much weight. I know you're trying, but you're making a mistake somewhere. You've already gained twenty pounds and you're only halfway through your pregnancy. At this rate, you'll gain at least forty to fifty pounds by the time you deliver. What's the trouble?"

"I don't know what is it, doctor, because I'm not eating anything."

"Well, you must be eating something."

"Maybe I *am* snacking more often."

"How many times do I have to say it, Joanne, you can't protect you or your baby with junk food! From now on I want you to eat only what I tell you to eat: lean meat, fish or poultry, green and leafy yellow vegetables, unsweetened juices and skim milk. I don't care how much of them you eat, but that's it. No potatoes or candy! No cakes or cookies! I want you to take your vitamins and minerals and get some exercise. You may drink as much as you wish, so long as it is only skim milk, unsweetened juices and low-calorie sodas—and, of course, abundant water. If you don't follow the rules, you may develop problems and we don't need that."

I've probably given that same lecture hundreds of times in the past twenty years. I gave the same advice to my patients who were not pregnant. A diet of high protein, low carbohydrate and fat works for both pregnant and non-pregnant women. I can be successful for you, and you don't have to be female either.

My pregnant patients were not on weight reducing diets. I wasn't trying to make them lose weight as much as I was trying to keep their weight under control and to keep them healthy. My main concern, then and now, was the health of my patients.

But many of my non-pregnant patients had serious medical problems because they were overweight. My first inclination, as you might have guessed, was to lecture them about the dangers of obesity. Unfortunately, they'd heard most of it before and it didn't have any effect.

So, instead of lecturing, I began recommending my diet to them. I told them the very same thing I told my pregnant patients. I explained to them that they didn't have to count calories if they followed my advice. They didn't have to measure their food. They didn't have to do anything out of the ordinary except to stick to the basics: lean meat, fish or poultry, green and yellow leafy vegetables and nothing more. I put very few limits on these foods.

I recommended my diet to overweight adolescents and to middle-aged women. For most of them, it worked beautifully. As I went along, I began to see fewer and fewer fat ladies coming into my office. I was tremendously pleased with this, because it meant my method worked. It also meant that my patients were becoming healthier.

The problem was that it didn't work for every one of them. For some, even a simple plan like mine proved to be too much. They just couldn't stop eating, no matter what. They could not control themselves. Most of them appeared to give up even before they got started. I think it was almost as frustrating for me as it was for them.

So I began looking for a way to make my diet easier. It was about this time that I became aware of the Protein-Sparing Modified Fast (PSMF). When I first heard of it, I thought that it might be exactly what I was looking for to help my overweight patients who couldn't seem to help themselves. As I learned more about it, however, I came to the conclusion it was *not*.

First of all, the PSMF was a very severe diet. It was so severe, in fact, that it was being administered only in hospitals and medical centers under strict medical supervision and it was being tried only on patients who were grossly overweight. Most of my patients did not fall into that category. Also, the PSMF called for eating nothing but predigested liquid protein, something that struck me as unnatural.

What would happen to people after they lost weight on the PSMF? I suspected they would go right back to the same self-destructive eating habits that caused the problem in the first place. It seemed to guarantee drastic weight loss, but there was nothing to insure that the dieter wouldn't gain it all back.

It seemed to me that the PSMF was not designed for someone who wanted to lose weight and still be able to live normally. It did not seem to be a diet that you could use at home, either. It struck me as being too severe for that.

But before I could make some kind of decision for myself, I had to know a bit more about predigested liquid protein.

Predigested liquid protein, I found out, is made from animal collagen which, in laymen's terms, is connective tissue, such as hide, tendons, and bones.

Hide? Yes, and the rest of the stuff that holds a cow together. These hides, tendons and bones are treated with various digestive enzymes, then gelatin, artificial flavoring and coloring is added, and there you have predigested liquid protein—a product of amino acids only.

That's it. While there may be nothing inherently harmful in it, it is not a nutritional supplement and it is not a healthful food substitute.

I also wondered how high a quality protein it was. All protein products are rated according to the PER, the Protein Energy Ratio. This rating system was devised by the Society of Analytical Chemists and is used as the standard by the U.S. Government to judge all other proteins.

The PER is similar to the government rating for meat —A, AA, Top Grade, etc. The protein used as the standard is casein, the protein contained in milk. It has all twenty-two amino acids, including the eight essential ones. It also has them all in the correct amounts.

Collagen, the protein source for predigested liquid protein, is not as complete a protein source as milk. It is not the same quality either. Casein is the standard.

The PER ratings are usually reported in plus or minus

figures. Milk protein is listed at + 2.7. Some of the pre-digested liquid proteins are reported as 0 or − .825, etc. The main difference between the two is obvious.

Chapter 18

P-86 Formula II

Even though I decided that the PSMF was not what I wanted to recommend to my patients, I was still looking for something that would make my diet more effective and easier to use.

That's when I was approached by Joe Harris, president of American Protein Products. He told me his company was manufacturing a *powdered* nutritional supplement called P-86. We discussed the various nutritional problems faced by dieters and I found that our philosophies were the same. Soon after our conversation, I was invited to become the company's medical director. I accepted.

Now, before we go any further, I know you didn't buy this book to read a commercial for P-86. I would be something less than honest if I didn't say this. I would also be less than honest if I told you P-86 was the only product of its kind on the market. It isn't. There are several other products similar but not identical to P-86.

When I became medical director for APP, I knew immediately that I wanted to make changes in the

97

formula. I knew that the original product fit into my weight control concept. I also knew it was very good. But I wasn't satisfied. I wanted to make it better.

For example, though the original formula contained high amounts of quality protein, it did not contain one hundred percent of the U.S. RDA of vitamins and minerals. This was very important. I wanted to create a nutritional supplement that would give the dieter *everything* he or she needed.

After six months of experimentation, and with the help of a food chemist, we produced P-86 Formula II. It still contains the highest quality protein available—milk protein—because it is the most natural to use. But it also contains a hundred percent of the U.S.RDA of vitamins and minerals.

P-86 Formula II is an almost perfect food. It is also simple to use. Since one tablespoon in one glass of skim milk taken twice a day provides you with eighty percent of your needed protein *and* all the daily requirements of vitamins and minerals, it's hard to make a mistake. When taken in addition to a well-balanced third meal, you get all of your daily nutritional requirements with an absolute minimum of calories, fat and carbonhydrate.

I have made some comparisons so you can see how my diet plan makes losing weight easy and successful. As you can see by the chart, three average meals with the usual assortment of snacks gives you: 3,744 calories; 189 grams protein; 37 grams fat; and 353 grams carbohydrate.

This would support a person weighing 250 pounds! The levels of all three nutrients are ridiculously high. But even this high level of protein cannot *guarantee* the right amount of those eight essential amino acids or the U.S.RDA of vitamins and minerals.

On the other hand, two meals of P-86 Formula II with skim milk plus one well-balanced meal gives: 1035 calories; 92 grams protein; 13 grams fat; and 108 grams carbohydrate. This means a calorie difference of 2,709 a day and translates into a weight loss of approximately five and one-half pounds a week. It also guarantees good nutrition.

Remember that the recommended daily allowance (U.S.RDA) of all three nutrients is 56 grams protein, 22 grams fat and only 100 grams carbohydrate. My diet puts you in line with these recommendations.

Three Average Meals

	Calories	Protein	Fat	Carbohydrates
Breakfast	420	16	6	76
Lunch	532.5	23.8	11	63
Dinner	2380	140	11	142
	3332.5	180	28	281
Evening Snacks (Average)	412	8	9	72.5
	3744.5	188.8	37	353.5

Three Average Meals (Lean)	Calories	Protein	Fat	Carbohydrates
	1757.5	94.1	32	217

Average Lean Third Meal	Calories	Protein	Fat	Carbohydrates
	765	54	11	80

Two P-86 Milk Drinks and One Average Meal (Lean)	Calories	Protein	Fat	Carbohydrates
	1035	92	13	108

Three Average Meals Detailed

Breakfast	Calories	Protein	Fat	Carbohydrates
Orange Juice (unsweetened)				
One cup	120	2	Trace	28
Corn Flakes & 8 oz. Skim-milk	$\frac{95}{100} > 195$	$\frac{2}{10} > 12$	$\frac{Trace}{1} > 1$	$\frac{21}{14} > 35$
White Bread				
1 Slice	70	2	1	13
Butter or				
Margarine, 1 pat	35	Trace	4	Trace
Coffee Unlimited				
	420	16	6	76

or: P-86 with 8 oz. Skim-milk	$\frac{35}{100} > 135$	$\frac{9}{10} > 19$	$\frac{0}{1} > 1$	$\frac{0}{14} > 14$

Lunch	Calories	Protein	Fat	Carbohydrates
Hamburger (lean)	235	19.8	9	23
Mustard				
(1 tsp. pouch)	5	Trace	Trace	Trace
Bun one	140	4	2	26
Pickle ½	2.5	Trace	Trace	Trace
Coffee Unlimited				
Beer, 12 oz.	150	0	0	14
	532.5	23.8	11	63

or: P-86 with 8 oz. Skim-milk	$\frac{35}{100} > 135$	$\frac{9}{10} > 19$	$\frac{0}{1} > 1$	$\frac{0}{14} > 14$

Dinner				
(Average)	Calories	Protein	Fat	Carbohydrates
Lean Meat, Fish, Fowl, 4 oz.	340	33	9	0
Vegetable, 2 Cups	220	16	Trace	38
Bread, 2 Slices	140	4	2	26
1 Orange	65	1	Trace	16
Coffee Unlimited				
	· · · · · (1757.5)			
Extra for Dinner				
Salad, 2 cups green	220	16	Trace	38
Cocktail 1½ oz. & 8 oz. Mixer	205	0	0	24
	2380	140	11	142

Evening Snacks	Calories	Protein	Fat	Carbohydrates
Pizza, 2 pieces	290	12	8	44
Beer, 12 oz.	150	0	0	14
	440	12	8	44
Peanut Butter Sandwich	234	8	10	48
Coke	150	0	0	39
	384	8	10	87
Average Values	412	8	9	72.5

The only thing the plan eliminates from your diet is extra calories.

It does this naturally. All the ingredients I selected for P-86 Formula II are from established food sources—milk, vitamins and minerals. There are no additives or preservatives. The beauty of the new formula is that you can eat comfortably, lose weight, get good nutrition, learn better eating habits and not count calories, because you're eating nothing in excess.

Not all powdered nutritional supplements are alike.

I know, because I spent a great deal of time researching the subject. I wanted to make P-86 Formula II the very best and I think I've succeeded. I would like to make a simple comparison between P-86 Formula II and another popular brand. Before we do that, however, we first have to learn a little bit about nutritional labeling.

The regulation of dietary supplements extends to labels. If, for instance, a product contains less than fifty percent of the U.S.RDA, it is not a dietary supplement and cannot advertise itself as such.

If it contains between fifty and one hundred and fifty percent of the U.S.RDA, then it is considered a dietary supplement and is required by law to provide a complete breakdown of its ingredients on the label. (Any product that contains more than one hundred and fifty percent of the U.S.RDA is considered a drug and must be sold as such.)

I want you to compare the P-86 Formula II label with the other label in the illustration. What are the percentages of U.S.RDA? Is it a dietary supplement? How much carbohydrate and fat does the other powdered product contain compared to P-86 Formula II? How many calories per serving?

If you will compare these labels, you will see that you would have to take twice as much of some of the other products to equal the nutrient value of P-86 Formula II. Some of the other products also contain fat and carbohydrate, which slow your weight loss by adding unnecessary calories to each serving.

Because of this, reading the label carefully is very important. I have seen products calling themselves "super" potent protein products or special "power" foods, but their labels tell a much different story. You should always look at the "Nutritional Information"

Nutritional Information

	Product 1 P-86 Formula II	Product 2 PVM	Product 3 SLIM-FAST	Product 4 NATURSLIM
Serving Size:	1 Tbsp.	2 measuring spoons	2 Tbsps. rounded	2 Tbsps.
Servings per can	56	22	16	22
EACH SERVING PROVIDES:				
Protein	9 gms.	17 gms.	5 gms.	17 gms.
Carbohydrate	0	0	20 gms.	1 gm.
Fat	0	1 gm.	1 gm.	0
Calories	35	80	105	70
PERCENT OF U.S.RDA—2 SERVINGS				
Vitamin A	100%	80%	40%	4% (or less)
C	100	100	50	4 (or less)
B_1	100	100	40	500
B_2	100	100	20	480
Niacinamide (Niacin)	100	100	50	200
Calcium	100	30	20	40
Iron	100	100	50	16
D_2	100	80	20	0
E	100	100	50	0
Folic Acid	100	100	50	0
B_6	100	100	40	200
B_{12}	100	100	20	0
Biotin	100	100	0	0
Pantothenic Acid	100	100	40	200
Phosphorus	100	40	20	0
Iodine	100	100	20	0
Magnesium	100	40	0	0
Copper	100	100	50	0
Zinc	100	100	40	0
Potassium	838 mgms.	70 mgms.	0	0
Weight of can	25 oz.	16 oz.	16 oz.	16 oz.

Note: The figures as listed above were in effect at the time this book was in preparation. Changes in formula or volume could be changed at any time by the manufacturer.

section of any label before buying the product. It must, by law, tell you its nutritional content per serving. I know of a product that has been fooling the public by calling itself a "power protein" when in reality it contains four times as much carbohydrate as protein! That means it is really a *sugar product!*

Also read over the list of ingredients for any product. Ingredients are listed in order of greatest weight by volume and will show you just how much of each substance the product contains. If they knew that, a lot of people could have avoided the sugar product I just mentioned.

Check the number of servings in each package. Compare the number of servings to the price. That way you can figure out how much each serving costs. On the previous page, I have created a chart so you can easily see the difference between the powdered products available.

Remember, be careful. Reading a label is not difficult, but it is important.

Chapter 19

Who Says Protein Is Bad?

The FDA has caused tremendous confusion lately by making public statements concerning protein and high protein diets, specifically the Protein Sparing Modified Fast (PSMF) which uses predigested liquid protein. Unfortunately, they've been making these highly critical statements before knowing all the details. To make matters worse, they have lumped all high protein diets together, an opinion that goes against all the facts.

The FDA was following up on "suspected" illnesses and deaths that they said were linked to the use of the predigested *liquid* protein. This is the FDA's job. In their enthusiasm to protect the public, however, the FDA failed to differentiate between the predigested liquid protein and *powdered nutritional supplements* like P-86 Formula II and others. They compounded this error by also failing to differentiate between the two types of diet —the PSMF, which eliminates eating altogether, and mine, which calls for sensible eating habits and good nutrition.

Because of this, people who were pleased with my diet and used it successfully were frightened away. They

105

were deprived of a healthy and safe approach to weight control and, most importantly, the right to make their own decision. The FDA made it sound as if both diets were the same and damned them all.

At the risk of repeating myself, let me state the facts as I see them:

Protein is essential for good health.

Weight is lost only by lowering calorie intake and *not* by eating high protein foods.

The PSMF is not the same as my diet. My diet calls for a relatively normal intake of food.

My diet is not a fasting diet. It is not a severe regimen.

Required Amounts of Protein Per Day*

Men (154 lb.)†	56 gm.
Women (128 lb.)†	46 gm.
Pregnancy, last 4½ mo.	(+30 gm.)
Lactation	(+20 gm.)
Infants	
0 to 6 mo.	Kg. × 2.2 gm.
6 to 12 mo.	Kg. × 2.0 gm.
Children	
1 to 3 yr.	23 gm.
4 to 6 yr.	30 gm.
7 to 10 yr.	36 gm.
Boys	
11 to 14 yr.	44 gm.
15 to 18 yr.	54 gm.
Girls	
11 to 14 yr.	44 gm.
15 to 18 yr.	48 gm.

* From Food and Nutrition Board, National Academy of Sciences–National Research Council: Recommended dietary allowances, ed. 8, Washington, D.C., 1974, The Academy.
† 0.422 gm. of protein per pound of ideal body weight.

Foods High in Protein

Food	Approximate Amount	Protein (gm.)
Beef, chuck roast	3 oz. cooked	23.4
Beef, hamburger	3 oz. cooked	20.5
Beef round	3 oz. cooked	24.7
Beef, club steak	4 oz. cooked	27.6
Lamb leg	3 oz. cooked	21.6
Liver (beef, calf, and pork)	3 oz. cooked	20.4
Pork loin	3 oz. cooked	20.7
Ham	3 oz. cooked	20.7
Veal, leg or shoulder	3 oz. cooked	25.2
Chicken	¼ broiler	22.4
Chicken, fryer	½ breast (4 oz. raw)	26.9
Chicken, hen, stewed	1 thigh or ½ breast	26.5
Duck, roasted	3 slices (3½ × 2¾ × ¼)	20.6
Goose, roasted	3 slices (3½ × 2¾ × ¼)	25.3
Turkey	3 slices (3½ × 2¾ × ¼)	27.8
Haddock	3 oz. cooked	20.2
Halibut	3 oz. cooked	21.0
Oysters	6 medium	15.1
Salmon	⅔ cup	20.5
Scallops	5 to 6 medium	23.8
Tuna	½ cup	15.9
Peanut butter	4 tbs.	15.9
Milk	1 cup	8.5
Cottage cheese	5 to 6 tbs.	19.5
American cheddar cheese	1 oz.	7.1

The PSMF diet was originally designed for use under hospital supervision and was specifically aimed at the morbidly obese. It was never designed for people with a minimal amount of weight to lose. My diet is recommended for those people who have only up to 20-25 pounds to lose. It is by far the safest, simplest way to lose that kind of weight.

My diet stresses not only good eating habits but also behavior modification, sensible exercise and good nutrition. Research has shown that this *total* approach to weight loss and weight control is the *only* successful way to lose weight and keep it off. Obviously, someone who has more than 25 pounds to lose will also do well with my diet plan.

Most Americans eat more protein than they really need, but no one ever died from eating too much protein, unless they had diseased kidneys or liver. If protein were inherently dangerous, we would have to outlaw meat, fish, poultry, soy beans, eggs and milk. Eating good foods doesn't kill.

Chapter 20

My Diet:
The Nutritionally
Supplemented
Diet Plan (N.S.D.P.)

I've said it before and I will say it again: Most diets lack a common sense base. Any diet—should be able to do two things simultaneously.

First, it should guard the health of the dieter and should help get his or her body back into nutritional balance. You should know that you're getting the essential nutrients—protein, vitamins and minerals— that you need to remain healthy.

Secondly, the diet should allow you to lose weight *rapidly*, and *steadily*, so that the loss reinforces your determination.

The diet should also be uncomplicated. A simple diet will encourage you to stay with it. No diet discipline is ever easy but we both know from experience how ridiculously difficult some diets can be. Mine is not one of them.

This is important: If you can't follow the diet and you give up, you're worse off than you were before because it reinforces the impression that you can't win.

Your new diet should teach you to re-think and change your own self-destructive eating habits, the underlying cause of your weight problem. In this respect, it should also give you a program of sensible exercise to follow.

My diet does all of this—the N.S.D.P.

It starts with the supplement. Two glasses of it with skim milk will give you the following: more than half of your protein need and all of your vitamins and minerals. By substituting a glass of the supplement for breakfast and one for lunch, you have eliminated the calories you would normally be taking in.

To complete the program, you eat one average meal a day. That meal, however, must consist of lean meat, fish or poultry, green and yellow leafy vegetables and, if you like, a salad. It should be an average meal. No oversized portions, no second helpings, no rich desserts, no extras. It may include a whole fruit and one or two slices of bread. It should be enough to satisfy your empty stomach but not your overindulgent appetite. (A meal of this size will be approximately 700-800 calories and will be low in carbohydrates and fats).

Why this third meal?

Eating is a natural process. It is *excessive* eating that is abnormal. This one meal allows you to control your food intake and still lead a relatively normal lifestyle. You don't have to become a recluse. You don't have to hide when your family sits down to eat dinner. It doesn't stop you from going out to eat with friends. It gives you the pleasure of eating, but restricts the amounts and types of food.

Eating is something to enjoy, and common sense will tell you that it's much easier not to eat during the day if you know you're allowed to have a good dinner. This one meal a day allows you to maintain a level of sanity while you're losing weight. You don't have to sit around sipping cups of bouillon or chomping on celery like a rabbit while others are enjoying their evening meal.

A complete fast is not necessary. It eliminates one of your most basic pleasures: chewing and eating food. A complete fast is unnatural and was developed mainly for people who are morbidly obese. Most people fall into what I would call a minimum weight loss category. They need to lose between fifteen and twenty-five pounds. My diet was specifically designed with those people in mind, as well as those who need to lose more.

My diet will help you to change your bad eating habits more easily and effectively. By eating one average meal a day, you are relearning the process of eating sensibly. The two glasses of the supplement are a healthful substitute for excess calories and, since you are limited to only one well-balanced meal, you don't have to spend half the day subtotaling your dinner. It gives you the chance to control the amount of calories you take in without worrying about them.

Now, in case anyone misunderstands: No diet—including my own—should be started without seeing your own family doctor first. I repeat: Do not even breathe deeply near a diet unless you have seen your own doctor. He knows you and he knows if you have any special problems that should be considered.

You should also consider setting a reasonable weight goal. Consult with your doctor and check your height and weight against the insurance tables. Don't be too eager to lose weight you may not have to lose.

Here's an example of what I mean. I recently received a call from a dancer who said she wanted to lose five pounds. Doesn't seem like much, does it? The woman in question weighed 110 pounds and stood 5′ 5″ tall. Despite the fact that she said weight was very important to her career, she did not have a weight problem. Losing those five pounds was completely unnecessary.

Don't be dumb about losing weight. Give it some thought first. Decide on a sensible amount of weight to lose and work toward that goal.

Chapter 21
My Diet (Cont.)

Since dieters often believe in magic, there is a tendency among them to chalk their weight loss up the effects of some "magic powder." This is sheer nonsense and something that will keep you from your goal. Magic won't help you, but understanding and common sense will.

The powdered supplement doesn't cause you to lose weight any more than the phases of the moon do. You do it yourself by restricting the type of food you take in. The supplement can help you to maintain good nutrition as a foundation, but it alone won't take any weight off. It is the carbohydrates and fats that will change your weight, depending on what you do with them.

On the average, you need approximately fifteen calories per day per pound to stay the way you are. If you weigh 250 pounds, for example, you need to eat 3,750 calories each day to maintain that weight. By using simple arithmetic, you can easily see what will happen if you restrict yourself to one small meal a day—a meal of less than a thousand calories.

You must lose weight. Since you are restricting carbohydrates and fats, your body will also begin to use its stored fat as a source of energy.

Practically all diets, including mine, rely on the restricted intake of carbohydrates and fats to achieve weight loss. The first low-carbohydrate diet dates back to 1863, when a London undertaker named William Banting published a book called A Letter on Corpulence Addressed to the Public. In it, Banting described how he lost 45 pounds over a period of several months by not eating what was then common English fare—bread, beer, potatoes and sugar. It was a huge success.

Banting's diet and most of the others that have followed since then have said the same thing—restrict or eliminate carbohydrates and fats from the diet.

As with most things, the question is one of degree.

What happens when you restrict your carbohydrate intake is as follows: Since the body uses carbohydrates as its prime source of fuel, the amount of carbohydrates in the diet also determines how much of the stored fat will be used for fuel. (Carbohydrates also act as protein protection—they keep the body from using its protein as fuel.)

Now, ketones are incompletely metabolized fats—on their way to becoming fatty acids—that are present in the system at all times. During a period of low carbohydrate intake, or none at all, the body produces more of these ketones as a source of fuel for the brain and central nervous system. This is called ketosis and it increases with the breakdown of stored fat for fuel. When that happens, you lose weight. The body uses both ketones and the broken down fat (in the form of fatty acids) as fuel.

Apparently this alternative fuel system is a biological throwback to a time in history when periodic starvation was commonplace. To protect itself from a lack of glucose, the body developed a mechanism to feed the brain and provide it with the energy that was missing in the diet. As year-round food production increased and periodic starvation declined, the body relied on ketosis less and less. But the mechanism did not completely disappear.

The problem with a severe state of ketosis is that the ketones may interfere with the passage of uric acid through the kidneys and a condition of acidosis may develop. (This may be partially controlled by drinking a reasonable amount of liquids.) For example, uncontrolled diabetes and complete fasting—without any intake of protein to protect the lean tissue—involve a severe state of ketosis. When this happens, the body also turns to the lean tissue for energy. This is a potentially lethal situation.

But, if the carbohydrate level is decreased rather than completely eliminated, the protein is protected and the body will still turn to its stored-up fat for energy. The ketone level will be raised, but not to an abnormal level. During any period of weight loss the ketone level will be above average.

The PSMF diet results in a severe state of ketosis. I cannot go along with it because it is completely unnecessary. My diet plan was designed to avoid severe ketosis because I've allowed for a normal amount of carbohydrate. My diet provide almost the normal value of approximately 108 grams of carbohydrate. (Average is 100 grams.)

Won't that slow your weight loss? Yes, but only slightly. I don't claim that my method is the fastest way to lose weight. I only claim that it's the safest and, in the long run, the most effective. It is not the slowest.

Chapter 22
Weight Loss

I can't guarantee the precise amount of your weight loss. If you've been overeating for years, it will be much harder for you to change your eating habits. Depending on how much weight you want to lose—and how much you weigh now—the rate of weight loss will vary.

There is no reason, however, why you can't lose as much as eight pounds a week. It is not unreasonable to lose twenty-five pounds a month with my diet. It's being done all the time by people who understand what they're doing and sticking to it.

Let's take a mythical 250-pound person who cuts her caloric intake from four thousand calories a day to less than a quarter of that. Each morning, instead of eating a heavy breakfast, she fills a glass with skim milk, puts in a tablespoon of the supplement and drinks it. Breakfast is out of the way. (Coffee or tea are perfectly okay in the morning as long as you cut out the cream and sugar.)

The same goes for lunch. A glass of skim milk and a tablespoon of the supplement.

Now, for the one meal of the day. We have chosen

dinner arbitrarily. You may find that eating during the middle of the day or later in the afternoon works best for you. There is no strict rule as to which meals you skip. For dinner she (our 250-pound woman) eats four to six ounces of lean meat, fish or poultry, a tossed salad and a vegetable. For dessert, she could have a slice of fresh melon or whole fruit. This is a sensible, well-balanced meal of less than one thousand calories.

Following this method, our 250-pound person will begin to lose weight almost immediately. She has cut her caloric intake, received all the nutrition she needs and still has had the pleasure of eating a full meal.

As her body adjusts to fewer carbohydrates and fats, it will also use its own stored fat as energy. This will increase the weight loss rate.

On the average, it requires 15 calories intake to maintain 1 pound of weight, therefore:

Weight in Lbs.	Average Calorie Need/Day
100	1500
110	1650
120	1800
130	1950
140	2100
150	2250
160	2400
170	2550
180	2700
190	2850
200	3000
250	3750
300	4500

But what of the person who has only ten pounds to lose? This person weighs, let's say, 145 pounds and wants to get down to 135. This is a very small weight difference. You need approximately 2,175 calories a day to maintain 145 pounds. At 135, you need 2,025 calories a day to maintain that weight. The actual caloric difference between the two weights is only 150 calories.

To lose that ten pounds may take time simply because the difference between the two weights is much smaller. This doesn't mean you're not losing weight. Far from it. Any time you restrict your calories to less than what you need each day, you will lose weight. It won't happen overnight. That is a medical fact you will have to learn to live with. You may actually see a change in measurement first. Then again, it could happen quickly.

Remember that everyone has approximately the same proportionate amount of lean body mass. In essence, then, we are all thin people.

You should not lose sight of that fact.

To lose 1 pound of weight requires a deficit of 3500 calories, therefore:

Calorie Decrease Per Day	Calorie Loss Per Week	Pounds Lost Per Week
500	3,500	1
1,000	7,000	2
1,500	10,500	3
2,000	14,000	4
2,500	17,500	5
3,000	21,000	6
3,500	24,500	7
4,000	28,000	8

Chapter 23

My Diet Without a Nutritional Supplement

"Why can't I diet your way without the nutritional supplement?"

Well, who said you couldn't?

My diet was originally designed without using a nutritional supplement and there is no reason why you can't do it that way. It requires an overall reduction in total caloric intake, something a great many dieters find difficult without some kind of help. I designed the supplement specifically to help you reduce the amount of calories in your diet and to provide you with the proper nutrition while you're doing it. If you think you have the will power to accomplish this without the supplement, go to it.

There are two methods of achieving your weight loss goal without the supplement. The first is by doing exactly what I did while I was a resident—simply restrict yourself to one regular, well-balanced meal a day. It should be high in protein and low in carbohydrates and fats. You should also be taking a vitamin and mineral supplement to make sure you're getting the right amount of nutrients.

I won't try to fool you—it takes a lot of will power to diet this way. You may find that it's easier to cheat.

Another variation—probably a better one—would be to replace the supplement twice a day with small meals consisting of lean meat, fish or poultry and/or vegetables, and then a lean, well-balanced third meal. The object in either case, is to restrict the amount of carbohydrates and fats.

Without the supplement, my diet requires a certain amount of self-control. That's why I created the nutritional supplement approach. It acts as a control agent until you've taken the right steps towards a new life style.

But, since self-control is the real goal of my diet, it may make more sense to you to try my method from the very start. I know it's difficult, but it's not impossible. Once you set your mind to it, nothing is impossible.

There are some things to keep in mind, however. First, be sure to see your doctor. He may have some helpful suggestions to make. Second, be sure to take a vitamin and mineral supplement to assure yourself of good nutrition. Third, try to adapt the diet to your own situation.

You may find, for instance, that eating one meal a day is not for you. You may want to break it up into three or four smaller meals. The secret is restricting your intake of carbohydrates and fats, not protein and to lower your caloric intake.

To achieve permanent weight control, you *must* change your attitude towards food and you must alter your life style. It can't be done in a day. Don't be hard on yourself if you fail. Most people need some kind of help.

Chapter 24

The Weight Loss Plateau

People often speak of reaching a dead stop during a period of weight loss. The realization that weight loss is not one long uninterrupted slide to slimness can cause depression and anxiety.

Why? Because they don't understand the weight loss process, and what people don't understand usually frightens and confuses them.

There is no need to be frightened or confused. If you are following my program correctly and have reduced your intake of calories, you are losing weight. All things being equal, there is no way you cannot be losing weight. Your scale may not reflect it as fast as you think it should but as long as you stick to the diet, your body will continue to use its stored fat for energy.

The phenomenon of the weight loss plateau works something like this: After you've lost a certain amount of weight—and this varies from individual to individual —your calorie needs become less. Remember, you require approximately fifteen calories a pound to maintain your weight. The less you weigh, the fewer calories you need. During weight loss, your calorie need is decreasing every

Unlimited Food List

VEGETABLES

Asparagus
Beets
Broccoli
Brussels sprouts
Cabbage
Cauliflower
Celery
Chard
Collards
Cucumbers
Dandelion greens
Escarole
Eggplant
Green beans

Kale
Lettuce
Mushrooms
Okra
Peppers (green or red)
Pickles
Radishes
Sauerkraut
Spinach
Squash
Tomatoes
Turnip greens
Watercress
Wax beans

DESSERTS AND FRUITS

Cranberries
Lemons
Gelatin, unsweetened

BEVERAGES

Beverages, artificially
  sweetened, containing
  less than 5 calories
  per 8 ounces
Bouillon
Clear broth
Coffee
Tea

JUICES (unsweetened)

Lemon juice
Tomato juice
Vegetable juice
All others, unsweetened

SEASONINGS

Flavorings
Herbs
Horseradish
Mustard

Salad dressing, less than
  2 calories per tbsp.
Spices
Vinegar

MISCELLANEOUS
Jelly, artificially
  sweetened
Sugar substitute

MEATS (6–9 oz.)
  Beef
    Steak—Filet
          T-Bone
          Sirloin
          Rump
    Roast
    Ground
    Corned
    Liver
    Kidney
    Bacon
  Lamb
    Chops
    Kidney
    Liver
  Pork
    Ham—Boiled
         Canned
    Chops
    Frankfurter
    Knockwurst
    Sausage
  Lunchmeats
  Veal

SEAFOOD (6–9 oz.)
  All
POULTRY (6–9 oz.)
  All

day because your weight is decreasing. As your weight decreases, your calorie deficit—the difference between what you need and what you're taking in—becomes smaller.

This has a direct effect on your actual rate of weight loss and accounts for the slowdown. As you get closer to your weight goal, the amount of weight lost each day becomes smaller. This is quite normal. Once again, this is because the difference between calorie need and calorie intake is so much greater at the beginning of the diet than at the end.

If you understand this, than you will also understand that a weight loss plateau means you're actually getting closer to your goal.

Occasionally, there is temporary water retention. But it is *temporary*. Your body will adjust itself and the effect will disappear in a few days.

This phenomenon of plateaus is nothing to worry about. It is completely natural. Ignore it and stick to your diet.

Chapter 25
Behavior Modification

Nutritionist Roger J. Williams calls it "body wisdom," and that has a nice sensible ring to it.

"Part of what is suggested by the phrase 'use your body wisdom,'" Williams wrote, "involves showing a certain amount of independence and choice in the selection of food. When one, for politeness or for other reasons, always eats whatever is set before him without discrimination, he is not using his body wisdom. When one knows and feels that one has had enough, and yet continues to eat just to be sociable or to please the hostess, one is not using his body wisdom."

What Williams means is simple. The body, the internal machine, knows when it's hungry. It sends this message: Feed me. On the other hand, the body knows when it has had enough. Then it sends an entirely different message: Stop feeding me. Even if you are feeding your body improperly—too little protein or whatever—the body has a habit of adjusting to the imbalance. Exactly how and to what degree isn't known yet, but the process of ketosis is a good example. The body knows what it needs and it will operate to get it.

127

A chronic overeater is a person who consciously or unconsciously ignores his or her own internal cues. The body yells for them to stop eating but they keep right on shoving food into their mouths. They pump themselves full of sugars and fats and that upsets the body even more. It then begins to produce more insulin to cope with the excess and that slows down the body's ability to metabolize excess fat. Then Big Eater's body wisdom is further put out of joint.

In the meantime, the gorger may be suffering from any number of vitamin and mineral deficiencies.

The chronic overeater is more responsive to external eating cues than to the internal ones. Studies done at a number of universities and research centers have reinforced this conclusion. An overeater will sit down after a large meal and consume a gallon of ice cream simply because it's there—even though his body is crying out to him to stop.

It would be great if more people were in touch with their body's cues. Our average overeater refuses to listen to anything but the siren song of his own jaws moving up and down.

For such people weight reduction without some kind of behavior modification is extremely difficult.

Adults

Before we get into techniques you can use to control your own behavior, you must consider your self-image. Too often people who are overweight suffer from a rotten self-image. They don't look good, they don't feel good, and people treat them like emotional cripples.

Remember all the times you visited the relatives and everybody pushed food on you by the truckload? "Eat, it's good for you," they said or "Go on, help yourself to another piece of pie." (This is what I call the Mama Syndrome.) These people are accessories in the crime of your overeating and they are dangerous. They simply reinforce the idea that you are a child and have no control over what you do. They mistakenly indulge your worst habits and by doing so, extend the misery that comes from being fat. More often than not, they do it out of misguided love and affection, and that makes it doubly hard to resist.

Starting here and now, you have to learn to say no!

I believe that we are all adults and that as adults we can make decisions. *You* are an adult. You are not a child. No one has to pamper you or indulge you or pretend they don't know how you look and how bad you feel.

You must develop a new self-image. This may sound simplistic. Don't worry about it. You have an image problem, and the only person who can change it is *you*.

No more of this I-Can't-Help-Myself foolishness. Adults can and do control their own lives every day of the week. For some reason or another, you missed out on the announcement—probably because you had your head in the refrigerator. Adults can change their life styles and can make lasting, important decisions for themselves. This is why they let adults run the world and not ten-year-old children. Children aren't expected to control themselves; adults, by definition, are expected to do just that.

Charting Your Own Behavior Patterns

After you've checked with your doctor about your diet, and he's given you the go ahead, take a one-week period and continue eating just as you have been. *But keep track of what you eat!* Write it down! The essential information you need is: *when* you eat, *what* you eat, *where* you eat, and *how you feel* at the time.

(This method has been used successfully by Smoke Enders to break people of another destructive habit. They are given a chart that goes right in the cigarette pack, and the smokers are instructed to mark down the times they smoke.)

Make up your own chart. Divide the day into hours to reflect your eating patterns. Don't skip a thing! Each time that refrigerator or cupboard door opens, you *must* write it down.

After a few days, your personal pattern will emerge. Did you eat when you were depressed? Did you have two bags of potato chips every day at three o'clock? Did you eat more by yourself or when other people were around? Did you eat late at night? Did you snack while watching television?

The purpose of this "eating" diary is to force you to become aware of your own pattern of eating. You are drawing your personal road map.

Your map may tell you things that you'd rather not know. If you don't have the strength to face your problem squarely, you'll try to avoid it.

Don't! The eating chart is there to help you. It may be a little depressing at first, but stay with it.

Once the chart is completed, study it. Learn where your problems are and take some positive steps to change them. If, for instance, you eat ice cream late at night, stop buying it. The process of behavior modification is difficult, but not particularly complex.

All you have to do is say "No." Say "No" to those late night snacks. Say "No" to eating when you're depressed. Say "No" to your neighbors when they give you twenty-five pounds of spareribs at the next picnic. Say "No" to keeping mountains of candy around the house.

The first step is just to say "No!" Say "No" to Big Macs, Whoppers, fried chicken, potato chips, ice cream, lemon meringue pie, fried oysters, pork sausage, french fries, peanut butter and jelly, fudge, baked beans, cookies, candy and soda.

Kiss junk food goodbye.

How Others Can Help You Say No

If you're like most dieters, you've tried and failed so many times that your family just sighs at mention of another diet. They shake their heads, look up at the ceiling, and then they pass you the mashed potatoes. You feel guilty while you empty half the bowl.

This time it's different. You've all ready shown yourself what you can do by keeping your food chart. That's a healthy start. If you're going to all the trouble of doing that, then you're going to pursue the rest of it too.

What you don't need now is a lot of people sitting around telling you how you're going to fail. You don't want emotional charity, either. You don't want a pep talk. You want understanding.

You want to be treated like an adult.

So tell them! Explain to your family and friends what you're doing and why you're doing it. Don't tell them in the kitchen or at the dinner table. Do it in a nice neutral setting. Ask them to consider your problem, what you're doing about it and what they can do to help. This may mean a sacrifice on their part. If their eating habits are as bad as most Americans—whether they're overweight or not—then you're probably doing them a favor by pointing out that the junk they're eating is bad for them, too.

The point I'm trying to make is this: No one is super-human. It's a very tough thing to change bad habits. Your family can help. But your weight is ultimately your own problem and you will have to solve it yourself.

Tricks of the Trade

Here are some simple tricks you can use to change bad eating habits into good ones.

When you eat, do nothing but eat. Don't pollute your eating environment with a lot of other activity. Don't watch television. Don't read a book. Don't associate eating with any other activity. In that way you cut out a lot of cues that caused you to overeat in the first place. Confine eating to one room in your house and don't eat anywhere else.

Stop eating badly. Cut out *all* junk food. Replace sugar with a non-sugar substitute. If you feel a compulsion to snack, direct it elsewhere. Go for a walk. Ride a bike. Chop a cord of wood.

Avoid temptation. Buy only the quantity of food you and your family can sensibly consume. Don't overbuy! If you're single, buy only what you need. Don't keep a bag of cookies around to stare at you in the off-hours. Stop buying candy. Avoid fast-food places. When you go out to dinner, tell the waiter not to bring bread to your table. Don't order dessert. If necessary, ask your date, or your family, not to eat desserts when you're around. Don't buy prepared food. It's easier not to eat something if you know you're going to have to prepare it yourself.

Avoid falling victim to your emotions. This is tough. Since you know from your food chart that you eat when you're depressed or emotionally upset, find other outlets for those emotions. One way is to write your emotions down and reflect on them. Emotions are much easier to deal with if you can see them in black and white. Try to channel your anxiety into something creative.

For example, let's say you were always interested in art, although you may know very little about it. All right. Instead of eating when you're depressed, visit a local museum. The idea is to find enjoyable alternatives to eating.

Be more active. One of the main problems of our society is that we're lulled into less activity. There are automobiles, elevators, escalators and dishwashers. Inventors seem to conspire to keep you overweight because they keep you off the active list. If you shop at a store a few blocks away, don't drive to it, walk. Take the stairs instead of the elevator. Instead of ordering your kids to rake the leaves or mow the grass, assist them.

Chapter 26
Exercise

In 1972, the President's Council on Physical Fitness commissioned a study of our attitudes towards exercise and fitness. They came up with some startling statistics:

- Almost half of the adults did not exercise.
- Slightly more than half (55 percent) did any exercise at all. But 57 percent said they thought they got enough exercise to keep themselves fit.
- Of the Americans who did exercise, almost forty-four million walked; eighteen million rode bikes, fourteen million swam, and another fourteen million did calisthenics.

Unless you've been hiding under a cultural rock since 1972, you know that exercise is a current craze. Ours is an age of jogging. Physical activity from tennis to rope jumping is touted as the new way to go.

The relationship between a sedentary (inactive) life style and problem weight has been well documented. More important: exercise in combination with a high protein/low carbohydrate/low fat diet can help control certain heart diseases such as chronic angina.

135

Overweight people, who are sedentary by nature, find climbing stairs a major effort. They have also devised a few myths to keep themselves from recognizing the importance of exercise.

The first one is that it takes enormous activity to burn calories. This is also called the I-Hate-to-Sweat Myth. Not true. It does not take an enormous effort to burn calories. Nor is the word exercise synonymous with over-exertion and strain. You do not need to beat yourself to death to benefit from exercise.

The second myth is that exercise increases your appetite. Wrong. Reasonably moderate exercise may frequently reduce your appetite and may actually help your body control itself better.

Then there's the If-I-Exercise-Too-Much-I'll-Drop-Dead Myth. If you do too much of anything, you run risks. If you smoke too much, drink too much, eat too much, or drive your car ninety miles an hour too much, you are taking foolish chances. No one suggests you overextend yourself exercising.

But, if you're overweight, your problem is *not enough* exercise. It isn't that you exercise too much.

One of the reasons your grandparents always looked so thin yet ate so much was because they worked off those extra calories. In addition to eating properly, they were not pampered by labor avoiding devices and too much leisure time.

The National Research Council found that inactive men can eat only as much as 2,300 calories a day without gaining weight. *Active men* can eat as much as 4,500 calories a day. The difference is exercise and activity.

Without some form of exercise, any method of weight control, even my method, will be less effective. Exercise will not merely use up some excessive calories but it will also help strengthen your cadiovascular system, it will increase your endurance and lessen your fatigue. It will improve your muscle tone. You will feel better.

This is not a myth. This is a fact.

Now, before you run out the door to tear up the sod, let's do one very important thing.

Talk to your own doctor about an exercise program. If you're over thirty-five, this is an absolute necessity. If you've never done much exercise, he can tell you how much you should do when you start. Let's face it, you're out of shape. No one expects you to run a four-minute mile. Intensive, highly strenuous exercise are not necessary and as a start could do you more harm than good.

Some mild exercise would be: Walking to the supermarket instead of driving. Using the stairs instead of the elevator. Almost anything more active than sitting. Once you accept the idea that being active is healthy and important to your weight control, you can move on to something else.

Well, you ask, just exactly how many calories will I use up? Jean Mayer, a widely known nutritionist, put it this way: "On the average, walking for an hour will use up between 100 and 300 more calories than just sitting still; bicycling, up to 500 calories; swimming and skating, up to 600; skiing, up to 900. If you are a *well-trained athlete* [my emphasis], rowing can get you up to a caloric expenditure of some 1,300 calories . . . an hour."

The first secret of exercise is that it should be done regularly. Secondly, you must use common sense at the beginning. Don't over-exert yourself, but don't under-exert yourself, either. Ask your doctor about it. Together you can work out a system that is right for you.

What Kind of Exercise Should You Do?

That depends on two things—what you like doing and what you're capable of doing. Obviously, if you're forty-five years old you are not a candidate for the Dallas Cowboys. You may think that jogging is boring. You may have always hated bicycles.

There is really no "best" exercise. Exercise, like weight control, is your own personal choice. Choose wisely. One doctor suggested thinking about what you enjoyed doing as a child. Another doctor who is deeply involved in exercise therapy in California suggests using the word "play" instead of the word "exercise." Exercise sounds too much like work to some people. Substituting the word "play" is a simple mental trick to make it more appealing.

The amount of time you have to spend on exercise will also help determine what kind is right for you. If you live in the city, that will also influence your choice. The amount of money you are willing to spend will also influence it.

Let's say you only have an hour a day to exercise and you don't want to spend a great deal of money doing it. You could jump rope, do calisthenics, take brisk walks, or simply run in place in the comfort of your own living room.

If you belong to the YMCA or the YWCA, you have a much wider choice of activity. It can be done either alone or with a group of people. You will also have the benefit of trained supervision.

Examples of Daily Energy Expenditures of Mature Women and Men In Light Occupations

Activity category	Time, h	Man, 150 lbs.		Woman, 130 lbs.	
		Rate, cal/min	Total, cal	Rate, cal/min	Total, cal
Sleeping, reclining	8	1.0–1.2	540	0.9–1.1	440
Very light Seated and standing activities, painting trades, auto and truck driving, laboratory work, typing, playing musical instruments, sewing, ironing	12	Up to 2.5	1300	Up to 2.0	900
Light Walking on level, 2.5–3 mi/h, tailoring, pressing, garage work, electrical trades, carpentry, restaurant trades, cannery workers, washing clothes, shopping with light load, golf, sailing, table tennis, volleyball	3	2.5–4.9	600	2.0–3.9	450
Moderate Walking 3.5–4mi/h, plastering, weeding and hoeing, loading and stacking bales, scrubbing floors, shopping with heavy load, cycling, skiing, tennis, dancing	1	5.0–7.4	300	4.0–5.9	240
Heavy Walking with load uphill, tree felling, work with pick and shovel, basketball, swimming, climbing, football	0	7.5–12.0		6.0–10.0	
Total	24		2740		2030

Source: Food and Nutrition Board, National Research Council.

Check Yourself—See Your Doctor

As I said before, your doctor can tell you what you can and cannot do. This is particularly important for overweight people who haven't done anything except move spoon to mouth for many years.

Beyond that, you can test your limits of endurance yourself. The easiest way is simply to take a walk. How soon do you begin to feel out of breath? How soon before you experience a pounding in your chest and head? As soon as you find out, stop. You've gone about as far as you can go for that day.

If you're overweight *and* out of shape, these symptoms should appear fairly rapidly. *If* they continue beyond temporary discomfort, check with your doctor again.

If your muscles and joints are sore the next day, then you also know just how far you can go. The secret of exercise is *regularity, not severity*. It will do you and your body no good to flog yourself on Monday and then skip out for the rest of the week. It's better to do thirty minutes a day, every day, than to go crazy one entire afternoon a week. The AMA recommends between thirty and sixty minutes a day as a minimum amount of exercise.

Regularity is especially important for overweight people. In a way, it is a behavior modification technique. That is, you are setting up a *good habit*—exercising—in place of a *bad habit*—eating too much. According to one study at a leading university, a half-hour a day of exercise can keep off almost twenty-six pounds a year.

Once you know how much you can handle, you can begin your exercise routine. Slowly. Don't expect to look or feel like Mr. America or one of Charlie's Angels in a week. Eventually—usually over a period of about three months but only if you do it regularly—you will begin to feel better and look better. That's the terrific part. If you keep it up, it will happen. Just like that.

With continued exercise you will find an increase in strength and endurance. The odd aches and pains will go away. You will experience less fatigue and less tension.

Chapter 27

Permanent Weight Control

The object of any diet is to effect *permanent* weight control. Permanent weight control is impossible without a sensible plan and the realization that weight control is a *life-long project*. You can't just lose weight and then shuffle off into the sunset. The price of permanent weight control is permanent vigilance.

Fortunately, with my method, you already have an edge. You have a "control" that can be used safely forever. It is not a fad or a fad diet. It is not something that is going to disappear from the scene. As a matter of fact, my method could become a permanent diet program for millions of people all over the world. The reason is that it works, and, as Baretta might say on the "tube," you can take that to the bank.

But what is as important as my nutrition program is the degree to which you learn how to control yourself. My method is an aid—needless to say, a very good one— but it cannot replace *you*. You are the most important part of any diet. How successful you are is directly related to how well you've learned to control your own behavior. Without that control, none of what I've said will take place. Behavior modification means better, more intelligent eating habits and a more active life style—the *total approach* I've been talking about.

The hardest part of any diet is permanent weight control, but it is loaded with incentives. First of all, let's go back to the mirror. If you've followed my method and you've lost the weight you wanted to lose, you are probably enjoying the change. You may have noticed it even without your mirror. Those oversized dresses are too big for you. You've had to take in all your pants. You don't hang over your chair at the office anymore. People are beginning to treat you like a human being again. You get complimented on how you look. You're proud of yourself again.

Okay, back to the mirror. There, now you see the person you were meant to be. The real you. You're slim. You look and feel healthy. You've got your muscle tone back.

Let's face it, you look like a million bucks. What more do you want? A house in St. Tropez? A Rolls-Royce?

I can tell you what you don't want: You don't want to go back to your old figure.

The best method of permanent weight control is the same as the best method of weight loss: common sense, good nutrition, a more active life style and, above all, the pleasure in accomplishing what you set out to do.

The greatest advantage in my method is that it is *flexible* and can be adjusted to individual needs. If, for instance, the weight you've lost is minimal—twenty pounds or less—you may not have to stick to the two-glasses-of-nutritional-supplement-one-meal-a-day-regimen.

By checking the height and weight chart, you know approximately what your weight range should be. Since you weigh less than before, you will obviously need *fewer* calories a day to maintain it. That certainly will be *more* than the 1000-calorie limit that I recommended for the initial weight loss.

You will find that you can keep your weight under control by substituting a light lunch for your second glass of the supplement. It may also mean that you can treat yourself to a little indulgence now and then.

It does *not mean* that you can go on binges. What it *does mean* is that, within reason, you'll be able to expand your diet.

Keep this phrase in mind: *There is no such thing as a Free Lunch.* If you overeat or begin eating the wrong foods again, you will pay for it.

Your own body wisdom and your bathroom scale will help you decide how much supplement (and how much food) you'll need to maintain your best weight. Your own body rhythms will to a great extent, dictate your permanent diet.

Remember: Listen to your body wisdom and let your scale be your guide!

I've found in my life what I can and cannot afford to eat. I like to eat. I enjoy it tremendously and, if I let myself go, I would turn into the Goodyear Blimp in about six months. So, I only allow myself one meal a day. The rest of the time when I feel hungry, I have a glass of P-86 or some celery, lettuce, etc. I know I'm getting the nutrition I need so I don't worry about my health or spend hours wondering if I'm harming myself. I know I'm not. Then, when I do eat that one meal I enjoy it because I know *it won't hurt me.* I'm keeping my caloric intake down to a reasonable level without a lot of suffering. When I do eat, I eat freely, and I don't feel guilty if I have a sweet dessert every now and then.

Should you keep track of how many calories you're

taking in? Only if it suits you. You should keep track of all the extras. That "extra" snack before bedtime or that "extra" helping of whatever. Avoid extras! It is too easy to lose track of how much you're eating. This is also known as the Little-Bit-More Syndrome. Remember, keep using the same sensible restraint you used before. Counting calories is boring. Understanding your behavior and practicing nutrition is better. If you take the time to learn what is in this book, you will know, almost instinctively, what is bad for you.

Your intake of carbohydrates and fats is bound to increase once you're through with the weight-loss part of my diet. This is understandable and nothing to panic about. Keep in mind a few things.

First, try to make sure that the carbohydrates and fats you do eat give you something extra—vitamins, minerals, and fiber. Angel food cake doesn't count. Also make sure you eat a higher proportion of unsaturated fats rather than the saturated kind. Switch from butter to margarine. Make sure you buy lean cuts of meat and trim the fat on those. Cut down on fast food, junk food and over-processed prepared food.

By concentrating on these points, you will be doing two things. One, you'll be buying a form of life insurance. Eating better means living better and probably longer. (Remember those Russians who live to be 110 years old?)

Another benefit will be saving money. Yes, saving money. By using a nutritional supplement for one or two meals a day, you won't be eating and you won't have to buy anything but the supplement. By cutting down on your food intake—particularly high-priced items like prepared dishes and expensive meats— you will be saving money. How much you save obviously depends on the diet that works best for you.

If you're a woman and you're a homemaker, you'll be spending less time in the kitchen, and this means having more time to spend on youreslf, your family and the things you like doing best.

This may be the most important benefit of all!

Chapter 28
Side Effects

With any kind of diet there will be some people who have side effects. Obviously, the *positive* side effects are the goal of any diet program: increased vigor, energy, lack of hunger, better eating habits and, ultimately, weight loss and permanent weight control.

On the other hand, for a minority there are negative side effects. With any change in eating habits, these effects are almost impossible to avoid. They may include headache, cramps, constipation or diarrhea. Under my program of eating at least one fully balanced meal a day, these effects are usually short-lived and disappear within a week to ten days.

(Other, more serious, side effects like gout, cardiac arhythmia, dehydration and hypothalemia [low potassium] are *not* the result of my diet. They are caused by the dieter not following the rules and overdoing the degree of fasting. My diet is not a severe diet—don't turn it into one!)

There are people who should be wary about starting any new diet. They include people on medication such as insulin, anti-hypertensives, and digitalis. These people need careful medical supervision and examination before and during the diet. Anyone on these drugs should not be on any kind of "do it yourself" diet without a specific okay from the doctor.

Also, people with psychiatric problems, particularly those with suicidal tendencies, should not diet without supervision. Anyone with liver, kidney or cerebral blood supply disorders may well be on a low calorie diet. But they should consult a doctor first.

What causes those minor side-effects, such as headaches and constipation?

No one knows for sure, but it appears that the decrease in carbohydrate consumption contributes to the loss of "quick energy" and occasionally to a feeling of light-headedness. This decrease in volume may also account for headaches, cramps and a change in bowel movements. Some side effects may be the result of the emotional changes that affect people while dieting.

All are temporary.

It never ceases to amaze me how often people blame common everyday ailments like headaches, diarrhea or constipation on "something" in their diet. I had a relative who, if he didn't have his regular visit to the bathroom every day, developed a severe headache. I could never convince him that it was all emotional. He just couldn't understand that he wasn't "ill" if he missed a bowel movement or two.

This also goes for a decrease in hunger. During the first days of the diet, you may experience a slight increase in hunger. After a few days, as your fat begins to metabolize, your hunger will fade.

There are basically two kinds of hunger. One is because your stomach is empty. The other is an appetite which is caused by the brain—a "false hunger." People too often succumb to their life style rather than their stomachs. We would all do a lot better if we listened only to our stomachs and not to our appetites. We might "desire" that extra piece of pie for dessert, but we don't really "want" or "need" it.

What should you do about these unpleasant side effects? When I have a headache or feel one coming on, I take one of the standard pills for relief such as aspirin or its equivalent. If I need a laxative, I try some bulk foods or one of the common laxatives on sale in the drugstore. Remember, also, a headache is a common occurrence and may have nothing to do with the diet.

If for some reason, you dont respond to such simple treatments, you should see your doctor. Often your symptoms are purely coincidental and have nothing to do with the diet program. If you've been following the rules, side effects should remain minimal.

It is also possible to be allergic to the milk protein in a supplement. If you are, you should not be using that particular supplement.

Don't stop drinking water. As long as your kidneys are normal, they will excrete the excess. Good health requires an adequate supply of liquids. With all diets, adequate water intake is essential.

There are those who will tell you they retain fluid. This may be true, but only under certain conditions. If someone has gained weight because of fluid retention, then something is dramatically wrong. Your kidneys excrete as much fluid as you take in, except for a small amount lost through perspiration and breathing. If your heart, liver or kidneys are not functioning properly, there is an excellent chance your body will swell—a condition called edema. This is a problem not related to my diet. See your doctor!

It isn't uncommon for women to feel "bloated" prior to or during their menstrual periods. Some women retain fluid when they are on oral contraceptives. This isn't unusual and is only a temporary condition.

Adequate liquid intake during any diet helps the dieter. Don't stop drinking any of the following liquids: water, low calorie soft drinks, and, tea and coffee, if you like. Remember, they won't hurt you and they will help you to reach your goal.

There is no one answer to the occasional problem of side effects. Everyone is different and individual reactions to the same diet will vary. I personally know of no one who has experienced severe side effects from my diet. The majority of people experience no unpleasant side effects at all.

Chapter 29

The Nutritional Problems of Children, Pregnant Women and the Elderly

There are those who claim that "children are little adults," but one thing is certain—they are "thinking people." They are concerned about their images, as attested to by the following poems.*

FAT

Fat is that, there is no cure
You sit and sit, while you are bored.
You sit there and sit there,
thinking of why you are fat.
But then you know,
that Fat is That!

T. S., Age 9

---

* From *Childhood Obesity*, edited by Platon J. Collipp, M.D. Copyright 1975 by Publishing Sciences Group, Acton, Mass.

REDUCED FROM FAT!

It's for your benefit
that you're doing it
to make you skinny
Reduced: from fat

So you do your best
It's a sort of a test
So you'll be happy
Reduced: from fat

So you want to try
I bet I know why
You want to get skinny
Reduced: from fat

Happy when skinny
and sad when fat
                    D. K., Age 12

WITH APOLOGIES TO DAVID

Strict is my diet; I must not want
It maketh me to lie down at night hungry
It leadeth me past the confectioners;
It trieth my willpower;
It leadeth me in the paths of starvation
    for my figure's sake

Yea, though I walk through the aisles of
    the pastry department,
I will buy no sweet rolls, for they
    are fattening;
The cakes and the pies they
    tempt me.

Before me is a table set with
  greens beans and lettuce;
I filleth my stomach with liquids;
My day's quota runneth over.

Surely calories and weight charts
  will follow me
All the days of my life.
And I shall dwell in fear of scales
  forever.
                          —Anon.

A CHILD'S CODE FOR DIETERS

I must lose weight
I will, I'll try
I must lose weight
I will not lie
I must lose weight
I know just why
And wave that ugly flab goodbye.
I envy those who don't have to try
I envy those who don't have to diet
I must lose weight
Oh God, I'll try
I must lose weight—
And I won't lie
                    —Z. K., Age 13

BRAND NEW
Feeling bad coz I was fat
Didn't know what to do
So I went on this diet
And I'm glad that I tried it.
Coz now I feel brand new!
          —J. C., Age 14
     (Lost 58 lbs. in 6 months)

There are certain groups of people for whom nutrition and weight control presents problems. Primarily, these people need an increased amount of protein, vitamins and minerals. In other words, they must be guaranteed good nutrition. In most cases, they are not dieting per se, but they do have to watch out for unnecessary and often dangerous weight gain. For them, the use of a nutritional supplement is worth considering.

But none of these people should be using any kind of supplement without certain guidelines.

1. They should not be on any kind of weight control program alone. This means see your doctor first and no do-it-yourself dieting.

2. The use of any nutritional supplement should be restricted to those who need guaranteed nutrition, not for weight loss alone.

3. These people should use a nutritional supplement only if it is recommended and supervised by their own doctor. A doctor can individualize any good supplement or program.

Children and Adolescents

Approximately ten percent of all children are obese and need to follow a healthy plan of nutrition and weight control. A nutritional supplement may be the answer. Too often, particularly in the case of adolescents, children are malnourished because they don't eat properly. There is intense social pressure to be thin which may lead them to try a "crash" type diet program.

Parents—with the advice and consent of their family physician—might want to explore the use of a nutritional supplement to guarantee good nutrition and to encourage sensible eating habits. Too often, kids eat high calorie snacks or junk food loaded with extra calories and fat. A nutritional supplement twice a day may help your overweight or obese child cut down on unwanted and unneeded calories. It will also make sure they get the right amount of protein, vitamins and minerals needed for good growth.

There are some things a concerned parents can do to help the overweight or obese child. The main thing is: Don't *overfeed your child*. Growth is not always continual and there will be periods when your child's growth pattern may start and stop. If during those periods a child doesn't feel like eating huge amounts of food, don't force him to do it.

You should encourage your child to be more active. Overweight or obese children tend to be less active by nature, and that contributes greatly to their weight problem, just as it will contribute to a weight problem in adults. Increased activity is an absolute necessity. If you're watching your weight, too, you might think about planning some activities together. That way, the child won't feel you're singling them out for some kind of "special" punishment. The best way to help the obese child is by your own good example.

Educate your children. Teach them about nutrition and exercise. Punishment for overeating is useless and destructive. Your child needs positive reinforcement, not punishment. Don't allow him to go on any "crash" diets. Instead, show a common sense approach to weight control, the same as you would for an adult.

Pregnant Women

It is my firm opinion—based on twenty years' experience helping pregnant women—that a diet high in natural protein, vitamins, minerals and low in carbohydrates and fats will be successful in producing a *healthful* weight gain during pregnancy.

During pregnancy, most women need as much as sixty percent more protein. They also need an increased amount of carbohydrates for energy and they must have at least 100 percent of their vitamin and mineral needs. Since they are literally feeding two people, this increased amount of carbohydrate should not contribute to an abnormal weight gain provided, of course, that the increased amount of carbohydrates is kept within reasonable limits.

Remember, the weight gain should be in the lean tissue of both mother and child, not fat tissue. Too often, pregnant women don't eat properly and become nutrition-poor, even though they are eating an increased amount of food.

In this case, a nutritional supplement may help by guaranteeing good nutrition and contributing to a healthy gain in lean body tissue by supplying the correct amount of amino acids.

This does not mean that pregnant or nursing mothers should diet. It means they should watch their weight carefully and keep it under control.

If you find yourself in a situation where you are gaining too much weight during pregnancy, then discuss the situation with your own doctor and ask him about the use of a nutritional supplement. Some doctors may not go along with their use and you should take your own doctor's advice.

The Elderly

What is "elderly?" Most nutritionists consider anyone over the age of sixty-five elderly and that usually means a change in life style and a change in eating habits. Past the age of sixty-five, the level of activity usually declines and the basal metabolism rate slows down somewhat. The process of nutritional absorption becomes less efficient especially in the case of protein, calcium and iron.

The elderly also need guaranteed nutrition.

An elderly person may also be susceptible to unwanted weight gain. Lean body mass may thin out slightly so the weight gain is usually a gain of fat tissue. Because of this, an increased amount of protein, vitamins and minerals is essential. A well-balanced meal plan, taking these factors into account, is absolutely necessary.

See your doctor first. Your seniority gives you no extra privileges or exemptions. See him before you start any kind of diet or supplemental food program. Weight control when you're older is a healthy practice provided that your vital organs—kidneys, liver, heart and digestive system—are in good condition.

Once cleared by your doctor, you will find that a nutritional supplement works in controlling your weight and providing the extra nutrition you need. But do not use any method of weight control or any nutritional supplement until you've seen your doctor.

Chapter 30

In Conclusion

Well, you have just finished reading another book about dieting—my book about my philosophy of weight control.

You might say "So what!" or "That made sense," or "Well, he certainly didn't waste words," or "This I have to try!"

If you say the first, good luck to you and I hope whatever method you use will be successful for you.

I hope, though, that you will say all of the remaining three statements.

I have tried to keep it as simple as possible. My philosophy of weight control *is* simple. I have presented a proven method of losing weight and thereafter controlling it by *doing* cetrain things—and by *not* doing others.

I have shown that weight loss and control *is* multiphasic—including sensible eating, proper exercise and learning a new eating lifestyle, with or without using a nutritional supplement.

I have shown that you do *not* have to count calories,

suffer, be frustrated or lose your mind or dignity while losing weight.

Please, feel free, at anytime, to write to me with problems or questions. I promise you an answer.

Goodbye and best wishes for great success in your program towards a thinner, healthier *new you.*

Frequently Asked Questions—in the Mail and in the Office

1. *Why is nutrition so important? I'm overweight, so how can I be suffering from malnutrition?*

You may not feel like you're suffering from malnutrition, my friend, but you certainly look like it. Malnutrition does not mean that you're starving or wasting away. It means you're not getting the right kind of nourishment, and being overweight is a sure sign that you're getting the wrong kind of nourishment. Your diet is full of sugar and too many calories, and it shows.

If you were getting the correct nutrition, you wouldn't be loading yourself up with all those extra calories. Good nutrition implies a balance. First, an energy balance—taking in only as many calories as your body can use, nothing extra. Secondly, a nutritional balance—taking in the right amount of vitamins, minerals and some of the healthier carbohydrates that give you more than just calories—like fiber.

By overindulging, you may be neglecting your protein intake and you may not be getting the correct amount of amino acids, something you need every single day. My diet is specifically designed to get your body back into nutritional balance and to keep it that way.

2. *Should I take a nutritional supplement any time I'm hungry or feel like snacking?*

You could, but that's not its purpose. A glass of P-86 Formula II in skim milk as a substitute for each of two meals will give you two-thirds of your protein needs and all of the vitamins and minerals you need to get through the day. It was not developed as a substitute for snacks, but it is healthier than junk food.

Junk food—those snacks filled with sugar—are a major part of your weight problem. Start learning to live without them. There are two ways to accomplish this feat. Find alternatives to snacking. Take a walk, read a book, or write a letter. Anything! Avoid watching the advertising on TV and in the newspapers during the day, and that may help you to ignore much of the snack advertising that is tempting you.

If you absolutely must snack during the day, severely restrict yourself as to the amount you eat and what you eat. Try nibbling on things like fresh vegetables or a single fruit.

3. *Isn't this just another fad diet? What's to keep me from getting fat all over again?*

There's no one on God's green earth to keep you from getting fat all over again, except you. Did you really expect to be told anything different? If you ignore the advice in this book and go back to old self-destructive eating patterns again, you'll get fat again.

This diet is not a fad diet, because it recognizes the

fact that quick weight loss alone is not the answer to long-term weight control. Weight loss is important. Weight control is important. But they are two entirely different things. That's why I keep insisting on a multi-discipline approach that emphasizes good nutrition, behavior modification, reasonable exercise, and, as an incentive to use these techniques, a weight loss method that is highly effective and safe. None of these will work if used alone. To be successful, you must use all of them together. *The Nutritionally Supplemented Diet Plan.*

4. If I follow your diet and begin losing weight, can I give myself a reward? A piece of pie or something like that?

Sure you could give yourself a reward. You could also go into a room and beat yourself with a stick. The question in both cases, is: Why would you want to? The reason you're on this diet is that you rewarded yourself a little too often. You gave yourself too many pieces of pie and now you're paying the price. Why encourage yourself to start all over again? Who needs the same old bad habits?

If you really want to reward yourself for sticking to the diet, then why not try something other than food. Train yourself to avoid overeating. Instead of a piece of pie or a bag of potato chips, take yourself to a movie. For a great many overweight people, food has become the center of their lives—they live only to eat. Thinking of rewards in terms of food only reinforces that attitude. Non-food rewards will help you to break that habit.

5. What happens if I haven't got the will power to stay on your diet?

The obvious answer is, you lose. But I believe that everyone has the power to do what is good for them. Simply because you haven't been able to find it in the past does not mean you won't ever find it. Learning to control your own life—in this case, your overeating—is something that *can be learned.* It's just a question of understanding a few simple techniques and applying them to your own personal situation. There's no magic involved and you don't have to be a superperson to do it. The secret is not to panic or get depressed.

Learn to relax. Learn to set realistic goals for yourself and then go about achieving those goals the best way you know how. Don't listen to a lot of fairy tales about being overweight—things like "Once a fatty, always a fatty" and other equally ridiculous notions. People who tell you things like that are wrong, and it's time you realized it. Besides, with my diet plan you have help. You can go back on the routine, using the supplement for one or two meals a day until your scale tells you to stop. Eventually you'll be able to do it completely on your own.

6. *How much weight can I really expect to lose on your diet?*

That depends on how much you want to lose. It also depends on your own individual metabolism, how well you follow the program and how carefully you relearn your eating habits. With my diet, you can lose up to five or more pounds a week or as much as twenty-five pounds a month. You could also lose less than that.

On top of this, weight loss is not always constant, and there will be times during my diet when your rate of loss will become slower. This is perfectly normal and nothing to get upset about. If you follow my instructions, you will lose the weight you want *and* you will learn how to keep it off.

Crash diets, the kind that claim you can lose twenty pounds in a week, are dangerous, unhealthful and unsuccessful in teaching you how to maintain permanent weight control. If you're only interested in losing weight fast and not interested in permanent weight control—or good nutrition—then go on a "crash diet." I'll see you in about six months when you wake up to find you still have a weight problem. I promise I won't tell you I told you so.

7. *Why can't I just skip my third meal and take P-86 instead?*

Because it's unsafe and unnatural not to eat food.

That's not how the diet was designed. The program works best when accompanied by one well-balanced meal. This meal gives you the additional nutrients you need, as well as a certain amount of fiber and bulk. You will have the satisfaction you want and not overburden your body with a lot of extra calories. This third meal also allows you to lead a reasonably normal life. I don't want you to avoid food completely, I want you to learn how to control your eating habits.

8. *What about drinking alcoholic beverages?*

Don't. They are high in calories and are a contributing factor to excessive weight gain (increased cholesterol, too!). Here's a partial list of the calories some alcoholic beverages contain:

A 12 oz. bottle of beer: 175 calories
A 4 oz. glass of egg nog punch: 335 calories

A regular Manhattan: 165 calories
A regular Old-Fashioned: 180 calories
A regular Tom Collins: 180 calories
A jigger of gin: 105 calories
A glass of sweet wine (Port) : 158 calories

9. *Why do I have to visit a doctor before I start this diet?*

For safety's sake. Your family doctor knows your medical history and can alert you to any special problems that have to be considered before going on *any* diet. Some people, such as those with chronic kidney or liver problems, may not be able to use this or any other diet. Your doctor will also be able to monitor your health and your progress during the diet. I suggest a monthly check-up to make sure that you're using my diet correctly.

10. *Why should I use this diet method? My sister lost weight just by counting calories.*

Then maybe that will be the best method for you. No one diet program is best for everybody. But everybody does need help and direction. Most people bounce from one diet to another without lasting success. My method will stop that if they will only try it.

Letters to Dr. Wechsler......

I receive a great many letters with queries about P-86 and my diet. Here is a cross-section of these letters and my responses to them.

I include them in this book because they are all authentic and so you can share the real experiences of others—many of which are most encouraging. (My publisher has the original letters on file at his office.)

Gentlemen:

I am writing in reference to the P-86 Formula II. I purchased a 25 oz. can with a friend of mine and we divided it in half. I was on it for approximately 10 days and lost approximately 4 lbs. I would like to continue the use of P-86 for a longer time period—maybe everyday as suggested in the instructions. But first I wonder if you could give me more information regarding the contents of the P-86.

Do *all* the ingredients come from NATURAL SOURCES? And are there any ingredients, even the smallest amount, that I should know about? I would appreciate it very much if someone would answer my questions honestly.

I am very interested, now more than ever, because I recommended P-86 to four of my friends who purchased it on my recommendation.

Thank you,
Mrs. C. A.

Answer:

The major protein of P-86 Formula II is a natural by-product of milk and there is nothing artificial added that I know of. The vitamins and minerals come from an approved laboratory. Don't confuse "natural" with "organic," however. "Organic" applies to produce—fruits and vegetables—grown without insecticides or chemical fertilizers. "Natural' means there are no "chemical" additives, such as preservatives. P-86 Formula II is a completely natural product.

Dear Sir:

In reference to your instant protein powder, please be advised that a very good friend of ours gave my wife some of your product and she found it superior to any other reducer used in the past. You see, my wife is an advanced diabetic and it is imperative that she remain on a very strict reducing program as per her doctor's orders. We have tried various health stores and pharmacies in the hope we may secure some of the P-86, but, to no avail.

Your product is the only thing effective and palatable enough to warrant the reducing program.

Respectfully,
Mr. D. E. P.

Answer:

I'm very glad, first of all, that your wife consulted her doctor about her weight problem. There should be no trouble using the P-86. In the future, I hope you have less trouble finding it.

Dear Sir:

I just purchased your P-86. I am inquiring if I can change the procedure. I have a digestive problem. I am supposed to eat more often then your plan requires. I am supposed to eat six times a day—small meals. I cannot take strenuous exercise and I only need to lose eight pounds. I am fifty-six years old.

I really would appreciate it if you could give me an answer to my questions.

Sincerely,
Mrs. L. F. C.

Answer:

I assume your "six small meals" a day were recommended by your doctor and, by all means, get his approval. The amount you eat should be based on his judgment and your satisfaction. I would suggest that you take the P-86 as you would ordinarily. But since you need to lose only a few pounds, I wonder if you really need to diet at all. Check carefully with your doctor. After all, his recommendations are the ones you need to follow.

Dear Sirs:

I wanted to let you know how pleased I am with your Protein "86". Over the past five years I have tried every diet available; Weight Watchers (two difference times), 1,000 calories a day, the one where you take needles every day and eat only 500 calories, Dr. Atkin's diet, etc., etc. and have been unable to stick with them long enough to lose enough weight to amount to anything.

I admit I almost gave up, but I was determined. The results have been great. My first aim was for twenty (20) pounds; then twenty-five (25); and on to thirty (30). After losing thirty-two (32) pounds, I have set my final goal for forty (40) pounds and that will be "it." Only eight (8) more to go and I will be satisfied. I have gone on "maintenance" off and on during the time I have been on your product to see if I gained back any weight, but the scale stayed the same.

Everyone I meet cannot get over the results. I feel so much better physically and mentally. I had been wearing some size eighteens (size sixteens if I didn't button the jackets) and am now down to a size twelve. My husband is as pleased as I am and the children are really proud of me.

Sincerely yours,
Mrs. W. C. S.

Answer:
Thank you, and congratulations!

Dear Sir:

JOY TO THE WORLD! ! !

A diet that really works! ! !

I had to write and let you know how great your P-86 Formula is for losing weight.

I started on it about a week ago and lost 7 pounds in 7 days. On most of the other diets I tried (and I've tried them all) I couldn't lose 7 pounds in 7 weeks! !

I really don't know how it works but I do know, from personal experience, that it does do the job.

I don't feel the least bit hungry between meals, and for someone who couldn't exist without cake, candy, ice cream, etc., it's nothing short of miraculous that I can walk by all the sweet and starchy items in the world and have not the slightest inclination to taste any of them.

I've still got a long way to go to reach my weight goal, but with a start like this, I haven't the slightest doubt that I can do it and reach the goal I'm aiming for.

I've had a little difficulty obtaining P-86—I can only get it in one store in my area, and sometimes they run out of it—but when they do have it, I buy several cans and have enough for several weeks.

I'd recommend it to anyone who wants a safe, quick way to lose weight, and some of my family has tried it and it's worked wonders for them.

Believe me, it's great—and I, for one, intend to keep on until I reach my goal.

Sincerely,
Mrs. H. M. R.

P.S.:   As suggested, I have P-86 in skimmed milk with ½ teaspoon of honey and ½ teaspoon of vanilla (and it tastes great) —and then a regular meal at dinnertime, and I don't feel any hunger pangs whatsoever.

Answer:

If you read this book, you will know why P-86 works and why most of the other diets don't. As for your lack of appetite, that feeling is exactly correct. What you are feeling is not a "miracle" but your body becoming more attuned to its own rhythm. Having gone off all the junk—"cake, candy, ice cream"—your body is thanking you. The half-teaspoon of honey strikes me as a nice touch, but don't go beyond the half-teaspoon!

Dear Sir:

My wife bought a can of your P-86 about a week ago and she seems to be having a little trouble with it. The first few days, she lost four pounds, but she hasn't lost any since then. As a matter of fact, she gained one pound back.

Your pamphlet isn't that detailed about the do's and don'ts. For example, what do you consider a balanced meal? Can you eat butter? Baked potatoes? Salad dressing? Is there an important reason for taking oil with it? She would really appreciate an answer.

She has been faithful to your diet, in case you might think she hasn't.

Thank you,
Mr. J. C.

Answer:

The process of weight loss is not always constant. People can lose from one to eight pounds a week. Neither is it uncommon for some people to reach a plateau where they see no immediate reduction in weight. Fluctuations like that are completely normal. This doesn't mean your wife should give up. If she's using the P-86 correctly and cutting her caloric intake, she will lose weight. It will take her longer than five days, however. Nothing happens after five days except the weekend.

A balanced meal consists of lean meat (non-greasy and non-fried) or fish or poultry, plus green and yellow vegetables. You should not eat bake potatoes. If you want to eat bread, it should not be more than two slices a day. No butter is allowed. Margarine can be used in its place. Drinks should include non-fat milk, unsweetened juices and diet soda. You may drink all the water, coffee, and tea you like.

Gentlemen:

Can you please supply me with the following information regarding your diet?

1. What do you consider a well-balanced meal?
2. Are potatoes and rice allowed at your meal?
3. How many slices of bread are allowed?
4. Is tea allowed? If so, can iced tea be drunk instead of diet soda?
5. Can unsweetened fruit juices and diet drinks, such as diet lemonade, be drunk instead of diet soda?
6. Can low-fat milk be taken in coffee?
7. Can butter or margarine be used on bread an in cooking?
8. Can a person with low blood sugar, thyroid condition or anemia go on the P-86 diet?
9. Can you have only one P-86 meal and one regular meal a day or do you have to have two P-86 meals in order to get the full benefit of the diet?

Your answers to these questions will be greatly appreciated.

Very truly yours,
Mrs. D. C.

Answer:

I'm happy to answer your questions. A balanced meal on my diet consists of lean meat, fish or poultry and green and yellow leafy vegetables. I don't recommend baked potatoes or rice. Bread is allowed, but no more than two slices a day. Tea, iced tea, unsweetened fruit juices, diet sodas, low fat milk and coffe are all perfectly acceptable.

Butter should not be used on bread or in cooking—substitute margarine on your bread. Yes, a person with any of these conditions can go on my diet, but *only* after getting the okay from their family physician first. Do not go on *any* diet without seeing your own doctor. To get the full benefit of my diet, you must have two P-86 meals a day.

Dear Sir:

I just tried your diet and I lost six pounds the first week. I feel good because I'm not hungry during the day. I have about eight more pounds to lose.

I would like to know, what kind of diet should I use after losing the weight I want? What should I do between meals if I want a cup of bouillon or a cup of Sanka? How much liquid should I take in? I'm afraid I'll just put my weight back on if I don't do it right.

Are we allowed to have cereal for breakfast once in awhile? Maybe these questions don't seem important to you, but when a person decides to lose weight, it's a big step.

Thank you,
Mrs. G. A.

Answer:

First things first. Weight control is a lifelong proposition. If you find that using P-86 twice a day with one full meal keeps you at the weight you want, then keep doing it. If you've modified the diet—say one glass of P-86 and two small meals, for example—and you find you're gaining weight, then you know you've made a mistake. Your scale will tell if your modified diet is working or not. Use your own judgment.

If a cup of bouillon or a cup of coffee doesn't add any weight then there's no reason not to drink them. Liquids, unless they contain sugar, won't add weight. Drink as much liquid as you normally would, just make sure it isn't the wrong kind of high-calorie liquid. Obviously chocolate milk, sweetened sodas and presweetened fruit juices are the wrong kinds of liquid for someone with a weight problem.

Gentlemen:

Several days ago, I purchased some P-86 Formula II. I am concerned with what I'm allowed to eat for my meal in the evening. I would appreciate it if you could send me a food list with the foods allowed.

For example, can I eat cottage cheese, cream cheese or butter on my slice of rye toast? What about potatoes, cheese, hot dogs, ketchup, mustard, mayonnaise, tuna or any other fish?

> Very truly yours,
> Ms. P. B.

Answer:

Cream cheese, butter, cheese, ketchup and mayonnaise are out. All contain sugar, saturated fats and empty calories. There is a list of foods you can and should eat enclosed with this letter.

Dear Sir:

I have been on your diet and it is fantastic. It is the best diet I have been on, and I've tried many. I'm not the least bit hungry during the day, so I don't want any snacks. In fact, I have eight other friends started on it. I just can't say enough about it.

I would like to ask a few questions. I'm taking birth control pills and I also smoke. I was wondering if that would affect my weight loss? I mean, would my taking the pill and smoking make me lose weight more slowly? I don't take any other medication and my health is good. I also exercise daily.

Sincerely,
Ms. M. D. S.

Answer:

Birth control pills and cigarettes won't affect the diet. The pills might make you feel a little bloated every now and then, but that has nothing to do with your weight. Cigarettes may give you cancer, emphysema and a heart attack, but they won't add any weight. The pill—particularly if you smoke cigarettes—may increase your chances of blood clots and heart attack, so you might consider finding another form of contraception. I'm very happy that you exercise everyday. I wish more people did.

Dear Sir:

Just a note to tell you I've been using your diet for two months and I've lost twenty-two pounds. I'm very pleased with it. I still have a long way to go, but I'm staying with it.

I want to mention that I'm sixty-two years old. My hair was gray and since I started on your diet, it is turning blonde again.

Sincerely,
Mrs. M. E. L.

Answer:

This is a letter I'm going to have framed and put on my office wall. I know of nothing in P-86 that will get rid of grey hair, but it sounds terrific just the same. Do blondes really have more fun?

Dear Dr. Wechsler:

Thank you for your letter and the complimentary can of P-86 Formula II.

I am very happy to hear that you are still in business with this particular protein product.

I find the results of one or two meals with P-86 Formula II most satisfactory and I am pleased that I can lose the weight I need without too much effort. Although I have only lost 18 pounds since September, I am happy not to lose it too fast and I only have 10 to 15 pounds to go to attain my desired weight. I think what made it even better was when I did not gain back any of the lost weight during the one month I went off due to a cold and Christmas. It taught me something about discipline and watching what I was eating. I am happy to be on this for one and two meals a day!

Again thank you,
Ms. G. A. B.

Answer:

Thank you for your very kind letter. I am pleased that you are so successful. You have proven what I have been saying about our diet plan.

I have recently written a book about dieting and I am going to insert your letter into it so as to point out what can be done by people who pay attention to proper diet instructions and plans.

Nutrition Quiz

A knowledge of basic nutrition won't do you much good unless you can apply what you've learned to your own life. That is the purpose of this quiz—to make sure you understand nutrition and use that knowledge to combat your weight problem.

1. How has the American diet changed in the last few years? How have your own eating habits changed?

2. How does sugar contribute to bad nutrition? Why has heavily refined food added to our national weight problem?

3. How does the body use protein? Carbohydrate? Fat?

4. Which has more calories per gram: protein, carbohydrate, or fat? Which is the most efficient fuel? Which is the least efficient?

5. What is "junk" food? When was the last time you ate some?

6. Bad nutrition contributes to which diseases? Which diseases can good nutrition help prevent?

7. What is the correct answer to the following statement? Americans eat too much a) sugar; b) saturated fats; c) protein; d) fiber.

8. The major factors in excessive weight gain are a) lack of regular exercise; b) eating too much; c) eating the wrong kinds of food; d) drinking too much beer.

9. Describe the things that contributed to your own weight problem.

10. List all the food items in your kitchen that contain sugar. List all the items that contain no sugar. When was the last time you ate either one of them?

Answers to the Nutrition Quiz

1. Our consumption of sugar has skyrocketed, while our consumption of more complex carbohydrates and vitamins/minerals has been decreasing. Our consumption of saturated fats found in all red meats is also increasing. We gobble meat at an astonishing rate, despite the high prices and the dangers of saturated fats and cholesterol. You should try to relate these trends to your own eating habits and try to figure out some reasonable alternatives at the same time.

2. Sugar provides the body with nothing but energy. It doesn't provide any vitamins or minerals or help strengthen your muscles or tissue. It may actually cause some vitamin deficiencies. On top of everything else, it is probably the biggest contributor to excess weight.

Refined or highly processed packaged foods contain sugar. Some breakfast cereals are as much as fifty percent sugar. Most of the sugar in refined foods is hidden. They don't tell you on the label or in their advertising, either.

3 and 4. The body uses protein to build lean tissue. The body must have a certain amount of protein every day, particularly the eight essential amino acids. If even one of those amino acids is missing, the process of tissue building will be incomplete.

Carbohydrate is the body's main source of quick energy. When carbohydrates are digested they are changed into glucose, which is the fuel unit needed to run your system.

Fats are highly concentrated energy and have twice the calories of carbohydrate. The body uses fat as a source of stored energy rather than quick energy. Fat is stored in the adipose cells, cells designed specifically for that purpose.

Keep in mind that the body has an energy balance. If you eat too much of anything—carbohydrate or fat—the body will convert the excess into fat tissue and store it away in the adipose cells.

5. "Junk" food is just that, junk. It usually contains empty calories and not much else. It is usually flavored and textured artificially with chemicals.

When *was* the last time you had some junk food?

6. Pick almost any disease and malnutrition contributes to it, because malnutrition (bad nutrition) is an abnormal state. It means your body's metabolism is unbalanced. Good nutrition means it's a balanced system and may help prevent as many diseases as malnutrition helps aggravate.

7. The answer is sugar and saturated fats.

8. All four of them.

9 and 10. For this you're on your own. Don't shy away from the questions, however. Dealing with them objectively can only help you understand why you're having so much trouble with your weight.